Ken C. Winters
Editor

Adolescent Substance Abuse: New Frontiers in Assessment

Adolescent Substance Abuse: New Frontiers in Assessment has been co-published simultaneously as *Journal of Child & Adolescent Substance Abuse,* Volume 16, Number 1 2006.

Pre-publication
REVIEWS,
COMMENTARIES,
EVALUATIONS . . .

"**D**r. Ken Winters has assembled A STELLAR GROUP OF AUTHOR-INVESTIGATORS. Too often, the empirical literature and research focuses on identifying risk factors for the development of substance abuse problems or on clinical trials testing treatment modalities at the expense of developing a literature on assessment. This book fills that void quite nicely. Other important topics include concordance among adolescent self-report, collateral reports, urine drug screens, comparison of anonymous surveys with confidential surveys of substance use, and an examination of gender differences within the context of the psychometric properties of the Personal Experience Inventory (PEI), a popular comprehensive assessment tool for adolescents with substance abuse problems. THE READER WILL BE REWARDED BY THE DEPTH AND RANGE."

Oscar G. Bukstein, MD, MPH
Associate Professor of Psychiatry
University of Pittsburgh

Adolescent Substance Abuse: New Frontiers in Assessment

Adolescent Substance Abuse: New Frontiers in Assessment has been co-published simultaneously as *Journal of Child & Adolescent Substance Abuse,* Volume 16, Number 1 2006.

Monographic Separates from the *Journal of Child & Adolescent Substance Abuse*™

For additional information on these and other Haworth Press titles, including descriptions, tables of contents, reviews, and prices, use the QuickSearch catalog at http://www.HaworthPress.com.

Adolescent Substance Abuse: New Frontiers in Assessment, edited by Ken C. Winters, PhD (Vol. 16, No. 1, 2006). *To adequately address the problem of adolescent substance abuse, valid assessment is vital.* Adolescent Substance Abuse: New Frontiers in Assessment *provides counselors and researchers with important new research on under-studied topics of alcohol and other drug use behaviors by adolescents. Experts in the field of drug abuse and adolescent health discuss the latest studies that reflect new directions in the assessment of adolescent drug abuse.*

Etiology of Substance Use Disorder in Children and Adolescents: Emerging Findings from the Center for Education and Drug Abuse Research, edited by Ralph E. Tarter, PhD, and Michael M. Vanyukov, PhD (Vol. 10, No. 4, 2001). *"The culmination of many years of seminal work conducted by Drs. Tarter and Vanyukov and their interdisciplinary team of researchers. A cohesive and comprehensive model for understanding interactions between genetic and socioenvironmental influences on propensity to substance abuse. As a package, this book is complete in updating the reader on the state of the art in drug abuse research. Unlike many books in this field, this book is truly interdisciplinary." (Diana Fishbein, PhD, Director, Transdisciplinary Behavioral Science Program, Research Triangle Institute, Rockville, Maryland)*

Nicotine Addiction Among Adolescents, edited by Eric F. Wagner, PhD (Vol. 9, No. 4, 2000). *Containing research and current theories,* Nicotine Addiction Among Adolescents *offers researchers and medical professionals insight into emerging practices and methods of treating nicotine addiction in adolescents and thus helps them stop smoking.*

The Etiology and Prevention of Drug Abuse Among Minority Youth, edited by Gilbert J. Botvin, PhD, and Steven Schinke, PhD (Vol. 6, No. 1, 1997). *"Provides information on the causes of drug use among minority adolescents, the strengths and limitations of different intervention approaches, and ways to work appropriately with at-risk minority teens." (American Public Welfare Association)*

Adolescent Substance Abuse:
New Frontiers in Assessment

Ken C. Winters, PhD
Editor

Adolescent Substance Abuse: New Frontiers in Assessment has been co-published simultaneously as *Journal of Child & Adolescent Substance Abuse,* Volume 16, Number 1 2006.

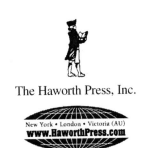

The Haworth Press, Inc.

New York • London • Victoria (AU)
www.HaworthPress.com

Adolescent Substance Abuse: New Frontiers in Assessment has been co-published simultaneously as *Journal of Child & Adolescent Substance Abuse*™, Volume 16, Number 1 2006.

Library of Congress Cataloging-in-Publication Data

Adolescent substance abuse : new frontiers in assessment / Ken C. Winters, editor.
    p. cm.
    "Co-published simultaneously as Journal of Child & Adolescent Substance Abuse, Volume 16, Number 1 2006."
    Includes bibliographical references and index.
    ISBN-13: 978-0-7890-3505-9 (hard cover : alk. paper)
    ISBN-10: 0-7890-3505-7 (hard cover : alk. paper)
    ISBN-13: 978-0-7890-3506-6 (soft cover : alk. paper)
    ISBN-10: 0-7890-3506-5 (soft cover : alk. paper)
    1. Teenagers–Substance use. 2. Teenagers–Drug use. 3. Substance abuse. I. Winters, Ken C.
HV4999.Y68A36 2007
362.29'12–dc22

2006029462

Indexing, Abstracting & Website/Internet Coverage

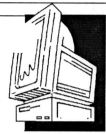

This section provides you with a list of major indexing & abstracting services and other tools for bibliographic access. That is to say, each service began covering this periodical during the year noted in the right column. Most Websites which are listed below have indicated that they will either post, disseminate, compile, archive, cite or alert their own Website users with research-based content from this work. (This list is as current as the copyright date of this publication.)

Abstracting, Website/Indexing Coverage . . . . Year When Coverage Began

- *Cabell's Directory of Publishing Opportunities in Psychology (Bibliographic Access)* <http://www.cabells.com> 2006

- *Cambridge Scientific Abstracts is a leading publisher of scientific information in print journals, online databases, CD-ROM and via the Internet <http://www.csa.com>* 2000

- *Child Welfare Information Gateway (formerly National Adoption Information Clearinghouse Documents Database, and formerly National Adoption Information Clearinghouse on Child Abuse & Neglect Information Documents Database)* <http://www.childwelfare.gov> 2006

- *CINAHL (Cumulative Index to Nursing & Allied Health Literature) (EBSCO) <http://www.cinahl.com>* 1994

- *Criminal Justice Abstracts (Sage)* 1990

- *Current Cites [Digital Libraries] [Electronic Publishing] [Multimedia & Hypermedia] [Networks & Networking] [General] <http://sunsite.berkeley.edu/CurrentCites/>* . . . . *

- *Current Contents/Social & Behavioral Sciences (Thomson Scientific) <http://www.isinet.com>* 1990

- *Drug Policy Information Clearinghouse* 1998

- *EBSCOhost Electronic Journals Service (EJS)* <http://ejournals.ebsco.com> 2001

(continued)

- *Education Research Product Family (EBSCO)* **2006**
- *Educational Research Abstracts (ERA) (online database)*
  <http://www.tandf.co.uk/era> **2002**
- *Elsevier Eflow-l* **2006**
- *Elsevier Scopus <http://www.info.scopus.com>* **2002**
- *EMCare (Elsevier) <http://www.elsevier.com>* **2006**
- *Environmental Sciences and Pollution Management*
  (Cambridge Scientific Abstracts) <http://www.csa.com> **2006**
- *ERIC Database (Education Resource Information Center)*
  <http://www.eric.ed.gov> **2004**
- *Family & Society Studies Worldwide (NISC USA)*
  <http://www.nisc.com> **1991**
- *Family Index Database <http://www.familyscholar.com>* **1995**
- *Google <http://www.google.com>* **2004**
- *Google Scholar <http://scholar.google.com>* **2004**
- *Haworth Document Delivery Center*
  <http://www.HaworthPress.com/journals/dds.asp> **1994**
- *HealthPromis* **1997**
- *Health & Safety Abstracts (Cambridge Scientific Abstracts)*
  <http://csa.com> **2006**
- *Index Guide to College Journals (core list compiled by*
  integrating 48 indexes frequently used to support
  undergraduate programs in small to medium-sized libraries) .. **1999**
- *Index to Periodical Articles Related to Law*
  <http://www.law.utexas.edu> **1990**
- *Injury Prevention Web <http://www.injurypreventionweb.org>* ...... *
- *International Bulletin of Bibliography on Education* **1992**
- *ISI Web of Science <http://www.isinet.com>* **2003**
- *Journal Citation Reports/Social Sciences Edition*
  (Thomson Scientific) <http://www.isinet.com> **2005**
- *Links@Ovid (via CrossRef targeted DOI links)*
  <http://www.ovid.com> **2005**
- *National Center for Chronic Disease Prevention & Health*
  Promotion (NCCDPHP) <http://chid.nih.gov> **1999**
- *National Criminal Justice Reference Service*
  <http://www.ncjrs.org> **1995**
- *Ovid Linksolver (OpenURL link resolver via CrossRef targeted*
  DOI links) <http://www.linksolver.com> **2005**

(continued)

- *Project MAINSTREAM*
  <http://www.projectmainstream.net> 2005
- *ProQuest Discovery <http://www.proquest.com>* 2006
- *Risk Abstracts (Cambridge Scientific Abstracts)*
  <http://csa.com>. 2006
- *ProQuest Research Library. Contents of this publication are
  indexed and abstracted in the ProQuest Research Library
  database (includes only abstracts. . .not full-text), available on
  ProQuest Information & Learning <http://www.proquest.com>* 2004
- *Psychological Abstracts (PsycINFO) <http://www.apa.org>* 1993
- *Referativnyi Zhurnal (Abstracts Journal of the All-Russian
  Institute of Scientific and Technical Information–in Russian)*
  <http://www.viniti.ru> 1992
- *Risk Abstracts (Cambridge Scientific Abstracts)*
  <http://csa.com>. 2006
- *SafetyLit <http://www.safetylit.org>*. 2004
- *Sage Family Studies Abstracts* 1995
- *ScienceDirect Navigator (Elsevier)*
  <http://www.info.sciencedirect.com>. 2002
- *Scopus (see instead Elsevier Scopus)*
  <http://www.info.scopus.com>. 2002
- *Social Sciences Citation Index (Thomson Scientific)*
  <http://www.isinet.com>. 1994
- *Social Scisearch (Thomson Scientific) <http://www.isinet.com>* . . 1994
- *Social Services Abstracts (Cambridge Scientific Abstracts)*
  <http://www.csa.com> 1997
- *Social Work Abstracts (NASW)*
  <http://www.silverplatter.com/catalog/swab.htm> 1990
- *Social Work Access Network (SWAN)*
  <http://cosw.sc.edu/swan/media.html> 2005
- *Sociological Abstracts (Cambridge Scientific Abstracts)*
  <http://www.csa.com> 1997
- *Special Educational Needs Abstracts* 1994
- *Studies on Women & Gender Abstracts*
  <http://www.tandf.co.uk/swa>. 1990
- *Ulrich's Periodicals Directory: International Periodicals
  Information Since 1932 (Bibliographic Access)*
  <http://www.Bowkerlink.com> 2006
- *Violence and Abuse Abstracts (Sage)*. 1994
- *Web of Science (Thomson Scientific) <http://www.isinet.com>* . . . 2003

*Exact start date to come

(continued)

Special Bibliographic Notes related to special journal issues (separates) and indexing/abstracting:

- indexing/abstracting services in this list will also cover material in any "separate" that is co-published simultaneously with Haworth's special thematic journal issue or DocuSerial. Indexing/abstracting usually covers material at the article/chapter level.
- monographic co-editions are intended for either non-subscribers or libraries which intend to purchase a second copy for their circulating collections.
- monographic co-editions are reported to all jobbers/wholesalers/approval plans. The source journal is listed as the "series" to assist the prevention of duplicate purchasing in the same manner utilized for books-in-series.
- to facilitate user/access services all indexing/abstracting services are encouraged to utilize the co-indexing entry note indicated at the bottom of the first page of each article/chapter/contribution.
- this is intended to assist a library user of any reference tool (whether print, electronic, online, or CD-ROM) to locate the monographic version if the library has purchased this version but not a subscription to the source journal.
- individual articles/chapters in any Haworth publication are also available through the Haworth Document Delivery Service (HDDS).

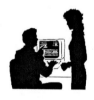

Adolescent Substance Abuse: New Frontiers in Assessment

CONTENTS

Introduction: Progress in the Assessment of Adolescent Drug Abuse   1
Ken C. Winters

Mapping the Clinical Complexities of Adolescents
with Substance Use Disorders: A Typological Study   5
Kathleen Meyers
Paul A. McDermott
Alicia Webb
Teresa A. Hagan

Community Readiness Survey: Norm Development
Using a Q-Sort Process   25
Anu Sharma
Andria M. Botzet
Rebecca A. J. Sechrist
Nikki Arthur
Ken C. Winters

Screening American Indian Youth for Referral
to Drug Abuse Prevention and Intervention Services   39
Ken C. Winters
Jerome DeWolfe
Donald Graham
Wehnona St. Cyr

Adolescent Alcohol and Marijuana Use: Concordance
Among Objective-, Self-, and Collateral-Reports   53
Joseph A. Burleson
Yifrah Kaminer

Adolescent Substance Abuse in Mexico, Puerto Rico
and the United States: Effect of Anonymous
versus Confidential Survey Formats   69
    William W. Latimer
    Megan S. O'Brien
    Marco A. Vasquez
    Maria Elena Medina-Mora
    Carlos F. Rios-Bedoya
    Leah J. Floyd

Gender Differences in Measuring Adolescent Drug Abuse
and Related Psychosocial Factors   91
    Andria M. Botzet
    Ken C. Winters
    Randy Stinchfield

Index   109

ABOUT THE EDITOR

Ken C. Winters, PhD, is Director of the Center for Adolescent Substance Abuse Research and Professor in the Department of Psychiatry at the University of Minnesota. He received his BA from the University of Minnesota and a PhD in Psychology (Clinical) from the State University of New York at Stony Brook. His primary research interest is the prevention and treatment of adolescent drug abuse. Dr. Winters has published numerous research articles in this area, and has received several research grants from the National Institute of Health and various foundations. He was the Lead Editor for two *Treatment Improvement Protocol Series* (# 31 and # 32) published by the Center for Substance Abuse Treatment (SAMHSA) that focused on adolescent drug abuse assessment and treatment. He is a consultant to many organizations, including the Hazelden Foundation, National Institute on Drug Abuse, Center for Substance Abuse Treatment, World Health Organization, and the Mentor Foundation (an international drug abuse prevention organization).

Introduction:
Progress in the Assessment
of Adolescent Drug Abuse

The past 20 years have been characterized by a rapid growth of research in the development of screening and assessment tools for measuring the extent and nature of adolescent drug use involvement and related problems (Lecesse & Waldron, 1994; Winters, 2003). These advances in the development and psychometric evaluation of questionnaires and interviews have contributed to several improvements in the field: user friendly features and rigorous psychometric evidence justify the use of such tools in a wide network of professionals with diverse training and background; important differences between adolescent and adult drug use and the development of substance use disorders have been pinpointed with greater clarity; distinguishing normative from severe-end drug use behaviors in subgroups is aided by the numerous tools that provide non-clinical and clinical normative data for several demographic groups (e.g., gender and age); the multiplicity of tools now provides a statistical basis for screening, referral and treatment planning; the detection of faking bad, faking good and other sources of compromised self-report are aided by response distortion scales; and comorbid conditions are measured with screens or comprehensive subscales.

[Haworth co-indexing entry note]: "Introduction: Progress in the Assessment of Adolescent Drug Abuse." Winters, Ken C. Co-published simultaneously in *Journal of Child & Adolescent Substance Abuse* (The Haworth Press, Inc.) Vol. 16, No. 1, 2006, pp. 1-4; and: *Adolescent Substance Abuse: New Frontiers in Assessment* (ed: Ken C. Winters) The Haworth Press, Inc., 2006, pp. 1-4. Single or multiple copies of this article are available for a fee from The Haworth Document Delivery Service [1-800-HAWORTH, 9:00 a.m. - 5:00 p.m. (EST). E-mail address: docdelivery@haworthpress.com].

THE NEED FOR MORE RESEARCH

But challenges remain. Adolescent assessment typically must be based more on self-report data than adult assessment and, thus, the validity of adolescent tools is vital. Adolescents have been shown to be inconsistent about their reported drug use when it comes to drugs used infrequently (Single, Kandel, & Johnson, 1975), and they tend to report greater past substance use and related problems at treatment completion compared to their reports at treatment intake (Stinchfield, Niforopulos, & Feder, 1994). The severity and course of adolescent is too short for biomarkers to be relevant (Allen et al., 2003), and parents can provide corroboration of only general drug use behaviors (Winters et al., 2000). Fortunately, some evidence supports the validity of adolescent self-report of alcohol and other drug problems: a large proportion of youth in drug treatment settings admit to use of alcohol and other drugs and associated problems and few treatment-seeking adolescents endorse questions that indicate blatant faking of responses (e.g., admit to the use of a fictitious drug); and the information provided by adolescents has shown general agreement with archival records (Kaminer, 1991). Nonetheless, a great deal more validity work is needed. Many tests do not report validity evidence as a function of race or ethnicity, and it is rare for test manuals or technical manuscripts to have examined its ability to measure clinical treatment outcomes (Stinchfield & Winters, 1997).

Other research needs are noteworthy. There is a lack of data as to whether current assessment tools can adequately identify several distinct levels along the problem severity continuum. It is unclear whether the distinction between substance abuse and substance dependence is diagnostically meaningful when applied to adolescents, and there is the need for more precise measures of the heterogeneous group of youth that meet criteria for abuse, particularly alcohol abuse (Martin & Winters, 1998). A related area is the need for more precise identification of related psychosocial problems that may contribute to the onset and maintenance of AOD involvement. Many existing tools assess psychosocial risk factors historically, which does not permit an understanding of the extent to which risk factors may precede the AOD use or be a consequence of it.

OVERVIEW OF THE SPECIAL VOLUME

The papers in this special volume provide examples of important new research on the assessment of alcohol and other drug use behaviors. The selection of articles was guided by my intent to show examples of how the field has matured. Thus, all selections represent research that addresses under-studied topics.

The paper by Meyers and her colleagues describe how assessment can be used to identify treatment-oriented typologies in order to improve treatment matching. Three profiles types were identified based on a range of client characteristics. Sharma and colleagues describe their research on filling an important instrumentation gap–the measurement of community readiness for drug abuse prevention. Her study describes validation data of the instrument. The paper by Winters and colleagues reports on the psychometric data of a screening tool used for problem identification and referral in American Indian populations. The remaining three papers address issues of the validity of assessment. Burleson and Kaminer describe the concordance of urinalysis, parent-report and self-report; Latimer and his colleagues examine international drug use survey data to see if anonymous and confidential surveys are comparable, a finding generally found in U.S. surveys; and Botzet and colleagues report a study on possible gender differences in measuring drug abuse and related problems.

REFERENCES

Allen, J. P., Sillanaukee, P., Strid, N., & Litten, R.Z. (2003). Biomarkers of heavy drinking (pp. 37-54). In J. Allen and M. Colombus (Eds.), *Assessing Alcohol Problems: A Guide for Clinicians and Researchers (2nd edition)*. Rockville, MD: National Institute on Alcohol Abuse and Alcoholism.

Kaminer, Y. (1994). *Adolescent substance abuse: A comprehensive guide to theory and practice*. New York: Plenum Publishing Corporation.

Leccese, M., & Waldron, H.B. (1994). Assessing adolescent substance use: A critique of current measurement instruments. *Journal of Substance Abuse Treatment, 11,* 553-563.

Martin, C.S., & Winters, K.C. (1998). Diagnosis and assessment of alcohol use disorders among adolescents. *Alcohol Health and Research World, 22,* 95-106.

Single, E., Kandel, D., & Johnson, B. D. (1975). The reliability and validity of drug use responses in a large-scale longitudinal survey. *Journal of Drug Issues, 5,* 426-443.

Stinchfield, R.D., Niforopulos, L., & Feder, S. (1994). Follow-up contact bias in adolescent substance abuse treatment outcome research. *Journal of Studies on Alcohol, 55,* 285-289.

Stinchfield, R.D., & Winters, K.C. (1997). Measuring change in adolescent drug misuse with the Personal Experience Inventory. *Substance Use and Misuse, 32,* 63-76.

Winters, K.C. (2003). Screening and assessing youth for drug involvement (pp. 101-124). In J. Allen and M. Colombus (Eds.), *Assessing Alcohol Problems: A*

Guide for Clinicians and Researchers (2nd edition). Rockville, MD: National Institute on Alcohol Abuse and Alcoholism.

Winters, K.C., Anderson, N., Bengston, P., Stinchfield, R.D., & Latimer, W.W. (2000). Development of a parent questionnaire for the assessment of adolescent drug abuse. *Journal of Psychoactive Drugs, 32*, 3-13.

Ken C. Winters

doi:10.1300/J029v16n01_01

Mapping the Clinical Complexities of Adolescents with Substance Use Disorders: A Typological Study

Kathleen Meyers
Paul A. McDermott
Alicia Webb
Teresa A. Hagan

SUMMARY. Because of the vast improvements in adolescent substance use assessment, it is widely recognized that adolescent substance

Kathleen Meyers is affiliated with the University of Pennsylvania School of Medicine, Department of Psychiatry, Center of Studies on Addiction, Instrument Development and Methods Center, Philadelphia, PA and Philadelphia Safe and Sound, Philadelphia, PA.

Paul A. McDermott is affiliated with University of Pennsylvania School of Medicine and Graduate School of Education, Philadelphia, PA.

Alicia Webb is affiliated with Temple University, Graduate School of Psychology, Philadelphia, PA and University of Pennsylvania School of Medicine and Graduate School of Education, Philadelphia, PA.

Teresa A. Hagan is affiliated with System Measures, Inc., Spring Mount, PA.

Address correspondence to: Kathleen Meyers, PhD, Philadelphia Safe and Sound, 1835 Market Street, 4th Floor, Philadelphia, PA 19103 (E-mail: kmeyers@phila safesound.org).

The authors thank Jeanne Frantz and William Tucker for assistance with data collection, Patty Fitzgerald for data entry and data base management and Ray Incmikoski for ongoing assistance throughout the Project.

This work was supported by NIDA grant # DA07705-06.

[Haworth co-indexing entry note]: "Mapping the Clinical Complexities of Adolescents with Substance Use Disorders: A Typological Study." Meyers, Kathleen et al. Co-published simultaneously in *Journal of Child & Adolescent Substance Abuse* (The Haworth Press, Inc.) Vol. 16, No. 1, 2006, pp. 5-24; and: *Adolescent Substance Abuse: New Frontiers in Assessment* (ed: Ken C. Winters) The Haworth Press, Inc., 2006, pp. 5-24. Single or multiple copies of this article are available for a fee from The Haworth Document Delivery Service [1-800-HAWORTH, 9:00 a.m. - 5:00 p.m. (EST). E-mail address: docdelivery@haworthpress.com].

use disorders (SUD) encompasses diverse drugs, patterns and etiologies and are characterized by extensive heterogeneity in other life domains. The next step in advancing adolescent SUD assessment is to classify adolescents with SUD into treatment-oriented typologies so that the question "What works with whom under what conditions?" can be empirically investigated. This paper: (1) identifies and describes seven subtypes of 205 adolescents with SUD in alcohol and other drug (AOD) treatment aged 12-18 years (via dimensions of delinquency, psychosocial problems, chemical dependency, and sexual risk behavior); and (2) examines whether certain patterns are distinctive among youth court-mandated to AOD treatment. Each profile type is described in terms of relative problem severity, prevalence for youth mandated to treatment through the courts, demographics, and performance on external measures of mental health and substance use disorders. Multiple logistic regression demonstrated that three profile types yielded 75.6% accuracy (sensitivity = 75.8%, specificity = 75.5%) for discrimination between court-mandated and non-court-mandated to treatment youth, even when controlled for the contributions of youth age, sex, and ethnicity. This paper discusses the need for triage to multiple treatments with varying levels of intensity for different subgroups of adolescents. If cost-effective services by setting by youth typology could be empirically identified and replicated, perhaps an *empirically-guided* cost-containment strategy would be developed and implemented by managed care and state government. In this way, the trend for a decline in the number and types of on-site services provided by AOD treatment programs might reverse, improving adolescent SUD outcomes. doi:10.1300/J029v16n01_02 *[Article copies available for a fee from The Haworth Document Delivery Service: 1-800-HAWORTH. E-mail address: <docdelivery@haworthpress.com> Website: <http://www.HaworthPress.com>* © 2006 by The Haworth Press, Inc. All rights reserved.]

KEYWORDS. Adolescent, drug abuse, assessment

INTRODUCTION

Vast improvements in adolescent substance use assessment have occurred over the past ten years. The number and type of adolescent-specific assessment instruments have grown, moving beyond simply assessing simple alcohol and other drug use (AOD) to assessing functional status in various life domains (see Winters & Stinchfield, 1995 for a review). Because of multidimensional assessment, it is now widely recognized that adolescent substance use disorders (SUD) encompasses diverse drugs, patterns and etiologies and are characterized by extensive heterogeneity in other life domains (e.g., behavioral, mood, environmental). The interaction of these life domains have been shown to influence treatment outcome (Loeber, Stouthamer-Loeber & White, 1999; Weinberg & Glantz, 1999) with treatment decisions for adolescents being better informed by pre-treatment psychosocial factors than drug use severity (Latimer, Newcomb, Winters & Stinchfield, 2000).

While these investigations indicate the need for multiple intervention approaches, adolescents are frequently treated with a single intervention approach within settings that fail to offer a wide and needed array of services (Delany, Broome, Flynn, & Fletcher, 2001; Dembo, 1995, 1996; Terry, VanderWaal, McBride, & Van Buren, 2000). The result? Many adolescents with SUD do not receive the type or amount of services to minimally address their needs (Delany, Broome, Flynn, & Fletcher, 2001), likely contributing to relapse and recidivism. Obviously, the severity of youth problems complicates treatment delivery and impacts treatment outcomes. Equally obvious, however, is the fact that substance abuse treatment programs cannot offer an exhaustive list of services and cannot be all things to all youth. Thus the question "What works with whom under what conditions?" continues to be posed (Winters, 1999), implying that there are interactions between types of youth and types of programs (Farabee, Sher, Hser, Grella, & Anglin, 2001; Riggs, Baker, Mikulich, Young & Crowley, 1995). The next step in advancing adolescent SUD assessment, therefore, is to classify adolescents with SUD into treatment-oriented typologies. Classification of other populations into various typologies has been shown to improve intervention effectiveness because they lead to better patient-treatment matching (see Jones & Harris, 1999 for work with delinquent youth; see Nurco, Hanlon, O'Grady, & Kinlock, 1997 for work with adult narcotic addicts; see Wieczorek & Miller, 1992 for work with DUI offenders).

Since multidimensional assessment of adolescent SUD has become the norm, the time is ripe to aggregate these data into a treatment-oriented classification system whereby prototypes of youth who share similar constellations of attributes would be empirically identified. Such a typological approach within adolescent SUD holds promise for: (1) designing and tailoring programmatic responses to the clinical complexities of this heterogeneous group of youth; (2) examining outcome trajectories with a particular focus on the identification of typologies that are related to the persistence and desistence of SUD (Loeber, Stouthamer-Loeber & White, 1999; Weinberg & Glantz, 1999);

and (3) formulating better developmental models of multi-problem youth. In this paper we explore whether different treatment-oriented typologies of adolescent SUD can be identified across various constellations of life domains. Because of the vast number of youth referred to AOD treatment programs by the juvenile justice system, we further explore whether any of the resultant typologies can distinguish youth court-mandated to AOD treatment from non-court-mandated youth.

METHOD

Participants

The full sample ($N = 205$) contained 126 males and 79 females aged 12-18 years ($M = 15.6$, $SD = 1.1$). Sixty percent of participants were White, 28% African American, and the remaining 12% from other ethnic groups (e.g., Asian-Pacific Islander). All participants were referred for substance dependence problems. Based on the relative length of dependence (in terms of years and months usage) for each type of drug, not including tobacco, 36.1% of the sample reported cannabis to be their primary addiction, 20.0% alcohol, 8.3% either opiates or cocaine, 5.4% barbiturates, 5.4% hallucinogens, and the remaining 24.9% a variety of less frequently used substances including amphetamines, inhalants, and over-the-counter drugs.

Whereas 67.8% of the youth were referred for treatment by health or welfare specialists, schools, family, or by their own election, 32.2% were mandated to AOD treatment directly by courts serving the juvenile justice system. This subsample contained 58 males and 8 females aged 14-18 years ($M = 16.2$, $SD = 1.0$). The subsample included 43.9% White youth, 40.9% African American, and 15.2% from rarer minority groups, with 50.0% reporting cannabis as their primary addiction, 19.6% alcohol, 9.1% opiates or cocaine, 7.6% barbiturates, 6.1% hallucinogens, and 7.6% other substances.

Measures

Comprehensive Adolescent Severity Inventory (CASI). The CASI (Meyers, Hagan, McDermott, Webb, Randell, & Frantz, 2006; Meyers, McLellan, Jaeger, & Pettinati, 1995; Meyers, Webb, Randall, McDermott, Mulvaney, Tucker, & McLellan, 1999) is composed of 10 modules, each focusing on a distinct area of adolescent adjustment:

health information, stressful life events, education, drug/alcohol use, use of free time, peer relationships, sexual behavior, family/household members, legal issues, and mental health. In turn, the modules contain 13 subscales that have been shown to retain appreciable internal consistency and to form four reliable and valid construct dimensions (Meyers et al., 2006). The Delinquency dimension is comprised of subscales assessing lifetime delinquent behavior, violent crime, nonviolent crime, and criminal justice involvement (63 items). The Psychosocial Problem dimension includes subscales on lifetime family problems, peer problems, and mental health treatment, as well as internalizing and externalizing disorders over the past year (142 items). The Chemical Dependency dimension assesses lifetime addictive behavior and drug and alcohol abuse (48 items) and the Sexual Risk Behavior dimension assesses lifetime sexual behavior and past year birth control usage (31 items).

General internal consistency for the dimensions ranges from .95-.86 and remains very high across subsamples by age level, sex, and ethnicity. Moreover, intraclass reliability over one-week is substantial and statistically significant for each dimension, with the percentage of reliable and uniquely interpretable variance associated distinctly with each dimension being substantial. The latent structure of the dimensions remains stable over age levels, sex, and ethnic subsamples, and the dimensions are shown to uniquely predict independent measures of mental health status, and drug usage one month and six months later.

Profile components. In the present study, each participant's profile was composed of his or her normalized T score ($M = 50, SD = 10$) on the four CASI dimensions. The T scores were derived through area conversion (Thorndike, 1982) such that identical scores across dimensions are associated with the same proportion of cases under the normal curve.

External criterion variables. The NIMH Diagnostic Interview Schedule for Children-Revised (DISC-IV) and Brief Symptom Inventory (BSI) were used as external validity criteria. The DISC is a fully structured interview for children and adolescents used to derive DSM-IV diagnoses (Shaffer, Fisher, & Lucas, 1997). For purposes of parsimony, the varied diagnoses are summarized under three composites: Internalizing diagnoses, Externalizing diagnoses, and Substance Abuse diagnoses. The BSI is a validated, self-report instrument that assesses mental health symptomotology (Derogatis & Spencer, 1982). BSI symptoms are summed under nine psychopathology dimensions. Both instruments have been subjected to extensive empirical verification and have been found to be reliable and valid.

Procedure

Data collection. Program staff explained study procedures to potential participants and their parent(s)/legal guardian(s) as a standard part of intake procedures. If parents(s)/legal guardian(s) agreed, written informed guardian consent and adolescent assent (including consent to be followed) were obtained. If time permitted, research staff were contacted and administered the baseline assessment battery (or scheduled an appointment for the assessment). A second assessment session was conducted approximately four days following the initial interview to assess test-retest reliability. One and six months post-treatment discharge follow-up interviews were also conducted as part of predictive validity procedures. Treatment completers and non-completers were followed. At each assessment session, interviewers administered the CASI and participants completed a battery of paper/pencil questionnaires. At the one- and six-month follow-up assessment sessions, biologic measures (i.e., urine specimens and breathalyzer readings) were also obtained. Detailed procedures can be found in Meyers, Hagan, McDermott, Webb, Randall, and Frantz (2006).

Typal development. The primary purpose of this research was the development and explication of a general typology of problems related to addiction severity. Our second goal was to assess whether the typology reveals distinguishing aspects of youth who are referred by juvenile justice systems. To this end, the 205 adolescent profiles from the four CASI dimensions (Delinquency, Psychosocial Functioning, Chemical Dependency, Sexual Risk Behavior) were sorted into mutually exclusive groups using cluster analytic procedures (see Meyers, Hagan, McDermott, Webb, Randall, & Frantz, 2006, for a description of these dimensions with component subscales). Cluster analysis was employed because it takes into account the complex nature of profiles, sorting them based on properties of level, shape, and dispersion. For the present investigation, profiles were sorted in such a manner to achieve typological distinctiveness, replicability, and full coverage. A three-stage clustering process was applied via computer program MEG (McDermott, 1998). First, the 205 CASI profiles were randomly partitioned into two mutually-exclusive blocks of 102 and 103 profiles, respectively. Ward's (1963) minimum-variance method was applied independently for the profiles comprising each block. For each block, the ideal number of clusters was determined through multiple criteria; specifically, (a) atypical decrease in overall between-cluster variance (R^2) and increase in within-cluster variance (Ward, 1963) with no reverse trend at subsequent steps, (b) ceiling of < 1.0 for the ratio of within-cluster variances to variance for the full supply of cases within each block, and (c) simultaneous elevation of the pseudo-F statistic (Calinski & Harabasz, 1974) over pseudo-t^2 statistic (Duda & Hart, 1973) as demonstrated by Cooper and Milligan (1988). (Note: Pseudo-F indicates separation among all clusters at the current step, whereas pseudo-t^2 indicates separation of the two clusters immediately joined at the current step.)

Clusters derived from the two independent first-stage analyses were pooled and subjected to second-stage clustering. Specifically, a similarity matrix was constructed to impart full first-stage history (cluster mean-profiles, radial and dispersion statistics, and within-cluster profile frequency) and Ward's method was reapplied. In this fashion, first-stage clusters provided independent replications of the final cluster solution. In addition, since agglomerative clustering provides no natural mechanism to relocate profiles retrospectively found to be misplaced, third-stage clustering applied divisive k-means iteration (as advised by Scheibler & Schneider, 1985) to relocate misplaced profiles.

Selection criteria for second- and third-stage clustering were identical to those in first-stage clustering and, in addition, several more conservative stopping rules were applied: Namely, (a) the average within-type homogeneity coefficient, H (Tryon & Bailey, 1970), must be $\geq .60$ (as per McDermott & Weiss, 1995), (b) the average between-types similarity coefficient, r_p (Cattell, 1949), must be < .40 (also see McDermott & Weiss, 1995), (c) each final cluster must have 100% replication rate as verified by absorption of first-stage cluster into the same second- and third-stage cluster (as per Overall & Magee, 1992), and (d) the solution must make psychological sense in terms of parsimonious coverage of the data and compatibility with relevant research on adolescent addiction.

Typal stability. Temporal stability of the typology was addressed using the profiles of a subsample ($n = 176$) of the full sample of 205 youth, where each member of the subsample also was administered the CASI one week after initial administration. As advised by Anderson (1986) and Perlman (1980), quadratic discriminant functions were applied to classify profiles from the one-week readministration based on the quadratic equations sensitive to profile levels, shapes, and dispersion within each profile type. Agreement between initial and subsequent classifications was evaluated using Fleiss's (1971) adaptation of coefficient κ. Overall κ indicated the short-term stability of the typology and partial κ assesses the temporal agreement of each specific cluster type.

Typal explication. Various internal and external variables were used to characterize and support the validity of the final typology. Level and pattern of cluster mean *T* scores were used to assist description of profile types. Deviations in the expected prevalence of age (where participants were divided into two groups; those 12-15 and those 16-18 years old, respectively), sex, ethnicity, and referral or no referral from the juvenile justice system within each profile type were determined by two-tailed tests of the standard error of proportional differences (Ferguson & Takane, 1989) for all pairwise comparisons across the criterion variable, with Type I error distributed across comparisons by the Bonferroni correction. Thus, interpretable prevalence trends for each profile type were based on statistically significant departures from full sample expectancy. Additionally, MANOVA was applied to identify significant interactions between the profile types and scores on the nine BSI dimensions and three DISC composites.

Finally, as a comprehensive test of the relevant factors distinguishing youth referred by the juvenile justice system from other youth, a multiple logistic regression model (Hosmer & Lemeshow, 2000) was developed where referral source (juvenile justice vs. other) served as the response variable, design variables reflecting the typology served as explanatory variables, and those demographic factors (age, sex, ethnicity) found pertinent at the prior research step served as control covariates.

RESULTS

Typal Structure

The first-stage analyses cumulatively produced 17 profile clusters. First-stage clusters were merged in a 17 × 17 similarity matrix and submitted to second-stage clustering. Having assessed each second-stage solution against the stated criteria, the seven-cluster solution was found superior and thereafter submitted to third-stage iteration to relocate misclassifications.

Table 1 shows that the seven-cluster solution satisfied all statistical requirements. It yielded impressive tightness-of-fit for profiles overall ($H = .83$) and within every cluster (range .92-.73) and appreciable separation between respective clusters ($r_p = .18$; range .33-.09), clearly ex-

TABLE 1. Prevalence, Homogeneity, Similarity, Replication Rate, and Reliability of the Typology of Adolescent Problem Severity

Profile type	% Prevalence	Within-type homogeneity (H)[a]	Between-type similarity (r_p)[b]	% Replicability across 2 independent blocks[c]	One-week classification stability (κ)[d]
Tp1	14.1	.92	.13	100.0	.79
Tp2	14.1	.87	.26	100.0	.56
Tp3	12.2	.83	.33	100.0	.70
Tp4	19.6	.81	.09	100.0	.69
Tp5	22.0	.77	.24	100.0	.69
Tp6	6.8	.87	.12	100.0	.81
Tp7	11.2	.73	.09	100.0	.62
M		.83[e]	.18[f]	100.0	

Note. N = 205. CASI = Comprehensive Adolescent Severity Index.
[a]Within-type homogeneity reveals the degree of profile similarity among the adolescents comprising each type. An *H* value of 1.0 would indicate that all adolescents within a given type have identical profiles. *H* decreases as the variability of profiles within a given type increases. An *H* of 0.0 would signify that the variability of profiles within a type equals the variability within the entire adolescent sample.
[b]Between-type similarity indicates the degree of similarity between the mean CASI profile for a given type and the mean profiles of all other types. An r_p of 1.0 would signify that the mean CASI profile for a type was identical to that of another type. As r_p decreases, the similarity between the average profile of a type and all others decreases.
[c]Replicability of every final type was determined by assessing whether it was found to exist within each of the first-stage cluster solutions. The percentage corresponds to the number of first-stage solutions in which each final type was found to emerge.
[d]Tests of statistical significance are based on Fleiss's (1971) formulae for partial κ assessing constancy of profile assignments over a one-week interval. *N* = 176 where all values are significant statistically at *p* < .0001.
[e]*H* is the mean of the within-type homogeneity values and is an index of the overall homogeneity of adolescents' profiles within the final types. Interpretation is similar to that of the *H* values described above.
[f]r_p is the mean of the between-type similarity values and is an index of the overall similarity (or dissimilarity) found among the average profiles of the final types. Interpretation is similar to that of the r_p values noted above.

ceeding the conventional $H \geq .60$ and $r_p < .40$ criteria. More notably, it produced perfect replication for every cluster across the two random blocks. Temporal stability for the typology (based on the one-week readministration sample) was 73.3%, a level 68.5% beyond chance (i.e., coefficient κ multiplied by 100) and statistically consequential ($p < .0001$). Moreover, partial κ values for each of the seven types was appreciable and statistically significant at $p < .0001$. No alternative cluster solution came close to meeting the requisite criteria.

Table 2 displays a descriptive name and corresponding mean *T* scores for each profile type. Note that the types are arranged in order of ascending problem severity with descriptive names based on the general level and shape of each prototypic (mean) profile. Tp2, 4, and 5 are distinguished by evidence for at least moderately severe delinquency, Tp3, 5, and 6 for at least moderately severe psychosocial functioning

TABLE 2. Descriptions and Mean T Scores for the Typology of Adolescent Problem Severity

Profile type	Descriptive name	Mean T-score profile			
		Delinquency	Psychosocial Problems	Chemical Dependency	Sexual Risk
Tp1	General Low Severity Problems	35	42	39	37
Tp2	Moderate Severity Delinquency and Chemical Dependency; Low Severity Psychosocial Problems and Sexual Risk Behavior	52	40	48	45
Tp3	Moderate Severity Psychosocial Problems and Sexual Risk Behavior; Low Severity Delinquency and Chemical Dependency	43	52	45	54
Tp4	High Severity Delinquency and Sexual Risk Behavior; Moderate Severity Chemical Dependency and Psychosocial Problems	57	48	52	60
Tp5	High Severity Psychosocial Problems and Delinquency; Moderate Severity Chemical Dependency and Sexual Risk Behavior	58	60	53	52
Tp6	Very High Severity Psychosocial Problems; Low Severity Chemical Dependency, Delinquency, Sexual Risk Behavior.	39	64	41	36
Tp7	Very High Severity Chemical Dependency; Moderate Severity Psychosocial Problems, Delinquency, Sexual Risk Behavior.	53	54	69	54

Note. N = 205.

(including mental health), and Tp2 and 7 for at least moderately severe chemical dependency problems.

Typal Explication

Table 3 summarizes the results of analyses to discover significant prevalence within profile types for youth juvenile justice referral, age, sex, and ethnicity. Tp1, the lowest severity type, is composed mainly of younger teenagers who were not referred through the courts. Tp3 youth are mainly females also not referred through the courts. In contrast, both Tp2 and 4, featuring moderately severe or higher delinquency, are primarily males who were referred through the justice system, with the more severe Tp4 also containing more African and fewer White youth than expected. Tp6, which represents the highest severity psychosocial problems, is predominantly female, whereas Tp7, the type featuring the most severe chemical dependency problems, is almost entirely comprised of older teens.

TABLE 3. Prevalence for Juvenile Justice Referral, Age, Sex, and Ethnicity Within the Typology of Adolescent Problem Severity

	Referral source		Age		Sex		Ethnicity		
	Juvenile justice	Other	12-15 years	16-18 years	Male	Female	Caucasian	African American	Other
Profile type	n = 66	n = 139	n = 89	n = 116	n = 126	n = 79	n = 123	n = 57	n = 25
Tp1	6.9	*93.1**	*82.8*****	17.2	51.7	48.3	51.7	34.5	13.8
Tp2	*65.5***	34.5	44.8	55.2	*93.1***	6.9	58.6	31.0	10.4
Tp3	4.0	*96.0***	60.0	40.0	28.0	*72.0***	72.0	20.0	8.0
Tp4	*57.5***	42.5	17.5	*82.5***	*92.5****	7.5	37.5	*45.0*a*	17.5
Tp5	33.3	66.7	40.0	60.0	57.8	42.2	62.2	22.2	15.6
Tp6	0.0	100.0	71.4	28.6	21.4	*78.6**	79.6	14.3	7.1
Tp7	26.1	73.9	8.7	*91.3***	47.8	52.2	82.6	13.0	4.4
Full sample	32.0	68.0	43.4	56.6	61.5	38.5	60.0	27.8	12.2

Note. Values are percentage prevalence where the row sum of values for each category (Juvenile justice, etc.) = 100.0. Tests of statistical significance are based on the standard error of proportional differences with correction for compound Type I error over multiple contrasts. Subgroups who dominate a profile type at a level greater than the expectancy established by the percentage for the full sample are italicized with $*p < .05$, $**p < .01$, $***p < .001$, or $****p < .0001$.
[a]Statistical significance refers to the test contrasting expected prevalence of African Americans versus Whites.

Tables 4 and 5 present typal trends with respect to the relative dominance of high scores on the various external criterion measures from the BSI and DISC. In general, Tp5 and 6, which convey the most severe levels of psychosocial functioning (including mental health), also tend to produce the most pathognomonic scores on independent measures of mental health. In turn, Tp7, which shows very severe chemical dependency levels, is often distinguished from Tp2 by more pathognomonic scores on external measures of mental health, Tp2 also representing chemical dependency problems, but with quite low levels of psychosocial problems. Consistent with its typal description featuring very high chemical dependency levels, Tp7 also is associated with more DISC substance abuse diagnoses.

Typal Discrimination

Given the evidence for the structure, stability, and validity of the typology, our second goal was to test the discriminatory power of the typology for distinguishing adolescents court-mandated to treatment versus those who were not court-mandated offenders from non-offenders. The foregoing analyses suggest that at least some of the profile types (Tp 2 and 4) have high prevalence for court-mandated youth and that this comports with the assertion of relatively severe delin-

TABLE 4. MANOVA Post Hoc Analyses for Dimensions of the Brief Symptom Inventory Across the Typology of Adolescent Severity

BSI dimension	Direction of typal mean differences[a]
Somatization	5 > 1, 2, 3, 4; 7 > 2
Obsessive Compulsive	5 > 1, 2, 4; 6, 7 > 1, 2; 3 > 2
Interpersonal Sensitivity	6 > 1, 2, 4; 5 > 1, 2
Depression	5, 6 > 1, 2, 4; 3 > 2
Anxiety	5, 7 > 1, 2, 4; 6 > 1, 2
Hostility	5 > 1, 2, 4
Phobic Anxiety	5 > 1, 2, 4
Paranoid Ideation	5 > 1, 2, 4; 3, 7 > 2
Psychoticism	5 > 1, 2, 4; 6 > 1, 2; 3, 7 > 2

Note. $N = 153$. Entries show which profile types differ significantly ($p < .05$ or better) and the direction of differences as based on Tukey's HSD test. The MANOVA effect for the interaction of the nine dimensions and seven profile types is $F(46, 688) = 2.09$, $p < .0001$, where Wilk's $\Lambda = .51$. BSI = Brief Symptom Inventory.

TABLE 5. MANOVA Post Hoc Analyses for Composites of the Diagnostic Interview Schedule for Children Across the Typology of Adolescent Severity

Composite area	Direction of typal mean differences[a]
DISC internalizing diagnoses	6 > 1, 2, 3, 4, 7
DISC externalizing diagnoses	5 > 1
DISC substance abuse diagnoses	7 > 1, 2, 4, 6; 5 > 1, 6; 3 > 1

Note. $N = 93$. Entries show which profile types differ significantly ($p < .05$ or better) and the direction of differences as based on Tukey's HSD test. The MANOVA effect for the interaction of the three composites and seven profile types is $F(12, 170) = 4.32$, $p < .0001$, where Wilk's $\Lambda = .59$. DISC = Diagnostic Interview Schedule for Children.

quency in their descriptive names–this prevalence for offending youth notwithstanding any peculiarities in the constituency of the full sample. But the analyses further reveal that prevalence trends for age, sex, and ethnicity also characterize those types and may alternatively explain why the types contain more offenders and why other types do not. Thus, separation of the competing theoretical networks, one favoring the typology and the other demographics, is required through a simultaneous multivariate treatment. To that end, multiple logistic regression was applied to predict court-mandated status, where age, sex, and ethnicity were forced into the model as control covariates and any or all of the profile types were permitted to enter the model as based on their ability to improve fit. Age was held as a continuous variable (i.e., 12-18 years) in order to provide maximum sensitivity to any changes in discriminatory power as youth aged, whereas sex was held as a binary design variable and ethnicity was represented by three binary design variables (Caucasian, African American, Other) with African American and Other entered into the equation and Caucasian held out as the contrast. The typology was represented by seven binary indicators (every participant scored 1 on the indicator corresponding with typal membership and 0 on the other six indicators), with the indicators for Tp2-Tp7 tested for model entry and that for Tp1 held out as the requisite contrast.

The resultant model is shown in Table 6 [$\chi^2(7) = 65.58$, $p < .001$, for the overall score statistic; area under the ROC curve = .85]. Discriminatory accuracy for the model was quite high (75.6%) with sensitivity and specificity (75.8% and 75.5%) illustrating comparable efficiency for identifying court-mandated and non-court-mandated adolescents with SUD. When controlled for the effects of other covariates, ethnicity

TABLE 6. Multiple Logistic Regression Model Predicting Juvenile Justice Referral Based on Demographics and the Typology of Adolescent Severity

Explanatory variable	Odds ratio	95% Wald confidence limit	
		Lower	Upper
Demography			
Age (12-18 years)	1.93***	1.82	2.82
Sex (Male)	3.18*	1.23	8.20
African American	2.00	0.88	4.56
Rarer minority	1.94	0.65	5.76
Severity type			
Tp2 Moderate Severity Delinquency and Chemical Dependency; Low Severity Psychosocial Problems and Sexual Risk Behavior	11.52****	3.53	37.03
Tp4 High Severity Delinquency and Sexual Risk Behavior; Moderate Severity Chemical Dependency and Psychosocial Problems	4.69**	1.64	13.36
Tp5 High Severity Psychosocial Problems and Delinquency; Moderate Severity Chemical Dependency and Sexual Risk Behavior	3.36*	1.23	9.15
Model chi-square[a]	65.58****		
df	7		
Goodness of fit[b]	.73		
% Classification accuracy[c]	75.60		

Note. N = 205. Entries are odds ratios expressing relative likelihood of juvenile justice referral associated with a given explanatory variable controlled for the alternative contributions of other explanatory variables in the model. Whereas the four demographic variables were forced into the model as control covariates, problem severity types were allowed to enter into the model only if model fit was improved significantly (i.e., Wald chi-square $p < .05$). The odds ratio for age indicates change in likelihood per each one-year age increment and ratios for other explanatory variables indicate likelihood when the respective characteristic is present.
[a]Inferential statistic assessing the significance of the overall model as per the score statistic.
[b]Probability level for the Hosmer-Lemeshow (2000) goodness-of-fit test, where nonsignificant values indicate plausibility of the model.
[c]Overall accuracy for identifying juvenile-justice referred adolescents versus other adolescents as based on conjoint maximum sensitivity and specificity levels.
$^*p < .05.$ $^{**}p < .01.$ $^{***}p < .001.$ $^{****}p < .0001.$

played no significant role in detecting court-mandated status, but the likelihood of court-mandated status increased on the average 83% with each additional year of life, while males manifested a greater than 3:1 odds over females for court-mandated status. Nonetheless, three of the profile types successfully improved the model after control for the demographic differences. Tp2 membership marked a risk for court-mandated status 11 1/2-times greater than types not in the model (as controlled for the alternative risk explained by Tp 4 and 5, which are in the model), and similarly, Tp4 membership affords a 4 2/3-times greater risk and Tp5 a 3 1/3-times greater risk. Noteworthy is the fact that the three types are the only types featuring high delinquency profiles. Tp5's discriminatory power is likely a function of its simultaneous covariation with Tp 2 and 4 in the model.

DISCUSSION

These results reflect the vast clinical and complex heterogeneity of adolescents in treatment for SUD. Using CASI data, seven treatment-oriented youth prototypes were empirically identified. These typologies were found to be stable and valid and discriminated court-mandated from non-court-mandated youth. As one reviews these typologies, vast clinical and research implications emerge.

Clinical Implications. At a most basic level, these seven typologies present AOD providers with the daunting task of delivering individualized intervention to such a diverse group of youth. While SUD may lead adolescents to treatment, there are equally severe and in many cases more severe life areas requiring intervention. Hence, treatment programs may be wise to develop different program tracks for different typologies, develop entirely different programs for different typologies, or restrict service delivery to the typology(ies) they are best at serving with referral of some typologies to other more appropriate services. These options could better insure that an array of services congruent with identified typologies would be available to accommodate and better address adolescent SUD heterogeneity. Admittedly, the reimbursement landscape could be a barrier to such an undertaking but a clinical-research collaborative could confront these challenges: Researchers track outcomes of typology by setting by services, thereby assisting clinicians with the development and justification for empirically-based program changes followed by subsequent reimbursement.

Within the triage process, these typologies may more thoroughly inform patient placement: matching youth to *type of setting* within an identified level of care. For example, while residential services (level of care) are indicated for TP7 and TP4 youth, these youth might be better treated in different "types" of residential settings. A traditional residential placement might be appropriate for the TP7 youth who is characterized by severe chemical dependency, while a therapeutic community as the residential placement might be a better match for the TP4 youth who has severe delinquency and moderate chemical dependency (Jainchill, Bhattacharya, & Yagelka, 1995; Jainchill, Hawke, DeLeon, & Yagelka, 2000). Taking placement one-step further, the use of these typologies could improve how one "selects" among similar settings within an identical level of care. For example, TP6 youth (predominately female adolescents characterized by high severity psychosocial problems and low severity chemical dependency, delinquency, and sexual risk behavior) might be best treated by an outpatient program that specializes in gender-specific programming, emphasizes the enhancement of psychosocial functioning and explores the use of drugs to modify negative mood states or stressful life events rather than being treated by a mixed-gender outpatient program that specializes exclusively in AOD treatment.

The emergence of the TP1 and TP7 typologies (i.e., youth who score low in severity across all dimensions, are young, and non-court-mandated; older youth with severe chemical dependency) takes interpretation, placement and treatment planning to another realm of clinical relevance. These typologies suggest that in addition to behavioral and drug use heterogeneity within adolescent SUD, there are developmental differences as well. This raises issues vis-à-vis the need for developmental tracks within adolescent-specific services or the need for separate programs for youth at different developmental stages and cognitive levels. While not entirely age-dependent, the approach to treatment might be very different for these two typologies due to reasoning abilities, egocentrism, etc. Further, according to Dishion and colleagues (Dishion, McCord, & Poulin, 1999; Poulin, Dishion & Burraston, 2001), "deviancy training" whereby problem peers negatively influence one another and reinforce problem behavior has been an unintended effect of their interventions and is most pronounced for younger adolescents. This not only calls into question the benefits of the group setting for these youth, but it further questions whether ages of adolescents should be taken into account during program selection, treatment placement, etc. If TP1 youth are more susceptible to "deviancy training," being grouped with older more severe adolescents might result in poorer outcomes, a similar unintended consequence found by Dishion.

With respect to youth court-mandated to drug treatment, three distinct profile types emerged: youth characterized by moderate delinquency, moderate chemical dependency, low psychosocial problems, low sexual risk behavior (TP2); youth characterized by severe delinquency, moderate chemical dependency, moderate psychosocial problems, severe sexual risk behavior (TP4); youth characterized by severe delinquency, moderate chemical dependency, severe psychosocial problems, moderate sexual risk behavior (TP5). These typologies could provide the legal system with an initial blueprint for differential placement and service provision (informed further by subsequent research) in the hope that offender-intervention matching would help to reduce recidivism and improve quality of life (McCord, Widom & Crowell, 2001). This line of inquiry is critical: (1) since, as the public health system reduces services, the juvenile justice system may find itself with more and more disordered delinquent youth (Mechanic, 1998) and little information on what to do with them; (2) if the juvenile justice system is to appropriately process, manage and intervene with these youth; and (3) if utilization of scarce resources is to be maximized. At a minimum, these results suggest that the judicial system needs to move beyond an almost exclusive focus on AOD issues to a broader focus on the multidimensional problems of these youth.

Research Implications. After tailoring programmatic responses to the clinical complexities of this heterogeneous group of youth, treatment-matching studies are indicated whereby youth with different typologies would be matched to settings and services/program tracks within a setting. These studies could begin to answer the question "what works best for which type of adolescent?" improving the capacity of the AOD treatment system to better meet the multidimensional needs of this heterogeneous population. Treatment-matching studies could then be followed by an investigation of the effect of typology on short-term and long-term outcome. These results could empirically inform the timing and duration of step-down services by typology since typologies that are related to the persistence and desistence of SUD will have been identified (e.g., "What minimum level of post-index treatment services are needed to maintain an 75% reduction in alcohol/drug use among TP 7 adolescents over the first year post-index treatment?"). Since certain co-morbid conditions follow different temporal courses (e.g., delinquent behaviors peak in mid-adolescence and decline in later adolescence; drug use rises throughout that period), it is possible that the temporal courses of different youth subgroups interact with one another, mediate or moderate overall and domain-specific outcomes, or confound outcome interpretation. Research to disentangle outcome trajectories by typology and treatment delivery could result in better developmental models of multi-problem youth.

In summary, these data illustrate the complex nature of adolescent SUD. While SUD may be the presenting problem, it is seldom the only problem or the most severe. Consequently, it is unlikely that improved functioning will involve a single intervention approach or that improved functioning will be quick, cheap, or easy (Winters, 1999). Instead, assessments that lead to the referral of different types of SUD youth to different types of treatments with varying levels of intensity will be necessary. Unfortunately, the best ways to match youth to optimal treatment approaches and the duration of these treatments are unknown, thereby requiring further investigation. If cost-effective services by setting by youth typology could be empirically identified and replicated, perhaps an *empirically-guided* cost-containment strategy would be developed and implemented by managed care and state government. In this way, the trend for a decline in the number and types of on-site services provided by AOD treatment programs might reverse (Etheridge, Hubbard, Anderson, Craddock, & Flynn, 1997), thereby improving treatment outcomes.

REFERENCES

Anderson, T. W. (1984). *An introduction to multivariate statistical analysis* (2nd ed.). New York: Wiley.

Calinski, T., & Harabasz, J. (1974). A dendrite method for cluster analysis. *Communications in Statistics, 3,* 1-27.

Cattell, R. B. (1949). r_p and other coefficients of pattern similarity. *Psychometrika, 14,* 279-298.

Cooper, M. C., & Milligan, G. W. (1988). *The effect of error on determining the number of clusters.* Proceedings of the International Workshop on Data Analysis, Decision Support, and Expert Knowledge Representation in Marketing and Related Areas of Research, 319-328.

Delany, P.J., Broome, K.M., Flynn, P.M., & Fletcher, B.W. (2001). Treatment service patterns and organizational structures: An analysis of programs in DATOS-A. *Journal of Adolescent Research, 16,* 590-607.

Derogatis, L.R., & Spencer, P.M. (1982). *Brief Symptom Inventory: Administration, scoring and procedures manual.* Baltimore: Clinical Psychometric Research.

Dishion, T.J., McCord, J., & Poulin, F. (1999). When interventions harm: Peer groups and problem behavior. *American Psychologist, 54:* 755-764.

Duda, R. O., & Hart, P. E. (1973). *Pattern classification and scene analysis.* New York: Wiley.

Etheridge, R.M., Hubbard, R.L., Anderson, J., Craddock, S.G., & Flynn, P. (1997). Treatment structure and program services in DATOS. *Psychology of Addictive Behaviors, 11,* 244-260.

Farabee, D., Shen, H., Hser, Y., Grella, C.E. & Anglin, M.D. (2001). The effect of drug treatment on criminal behavior among adolescents in DATOS-A. *Journal of Adolescent Research, 16,* 679-696.

Ferguson, G. A., & Takane, Y. (1988). *Statistical analyses in psychology and education* (6th ed.). New York: McGraw-Hill.

Fleiss, J. L. (1971). Measuring nominal scale agreement among many raters. *Psychological Bulletin, 76,* 378-382.

Hosmer, D. W., & Lemeshow, S. L. (2000). *Applied logistic regression* (2nd ed.). New York: Wiley-Interscience.

Jainchill, N., Bhattacharya, G., & Yagelka, J. (1995). Therapeutic communities for adolescents. In E. Rahdert & D. Czechowicz (eds.). *Adolescent Drug Abuse: Clinical Assessment and Therapeutic Interventions.* Rockville, MD. NIDA, 190-217.

Jainchill, N., Hawke, J., DeLeon, G. & Yagelka, J. (2000). Adolescents in therapeutic communities: One-year posttreatment outcomes. *Journal of Psychoactive Drugs, 32,* 81-94.

Jones, P.R. & Harris, P.W. (1999). Developing an empirically based typology of delinquent youth. *Journal of Quantitative Criminology, 15,* 251-276.

Latimer, W.W., Newcomb, M., Winters, K.C., & Stinchfield, R.D. (2000). Adolescent substance abuse treatment outcome: The role of substance abuse problem severity, psychosocial and treatment factors. *Journal of Consulting and Clinical Psychology, 68,* 684-696.

Loeber, R., Stouthamer-Loeber, M., & White, H.R. (1999). Developmental aspects of delinquency and internalizing problems and their association with persistent substance use between the ages of 7 and 18. *Journal of Clinical Child Psychology, 28,* 322-332.

McCord, J., Widom, C.S. & Crowell, N.A. (2001). Juvenile Crime, Juvenile Justice. Washington, DC: National Academy Press.

McDermott, P. A. (1998). MEG: Megacluster analytic strategy for multistage hierarchical grouping with relocations and replications. *Educational and Psychological Measurement, 58,* 677-686.

McDermott, P. A., & Weiss, R. V. (1995). A normative typology of healthy, subclinical, and clinical behavior styles among American children and adolescents. *Psychological Assessment, 7,* 162-170.

Meyers, K., Hagan, T. A., McDermott, P. A., Webb, A., Randell, M., & Frantz, J. (2006). Factor structure of the Comprehensive Adolescent Severity Inventory (CASI): Results of reliability, validity, and generality analyses. *American Journal of Drug and Alcohol Abuse, 32,* 287-310.

Meyers, K., McLellan, A. T., Jaeger, J. L., & Pettinati, H. M. (1995). The development of the Comprehensive Addiction Severity Index for Adolescents (CASI-A): An interview for assessing the multiple problems of adolescents. *Journal of Substance Abuse Treatment, 12,* 181-193.

Meyers, K., Webb, A., Randall, M., McDermott, P., Mulvaney, F., Tucker, W., & McLellan, A. T. (1999). Psychometric properties of the Comprehensive Adolescent Severity Inventory (CASI). *National Institute on Drug Abuse Research Monograph: Problems of Drug Dependence, Proceedings of the 60th Annual Scientific Meeting, College on Problems of Drug Dependence.*

Nurco, D.N., Hanlon, T.E., O'Grady, K.E., & Kinlock, T.W. (1997). The early emergence of narcotic addict subtypes. *American Journal of Drug and Alcohol Abuse, 23*, 523-542.

Overall, J. E., & Magee, K. N. (1992). Replication as a rule for determining the number of clusters in hierarchical cluster analysis. *Applied Psychological Measurement, 16*, 119-128.

Perlman, M. D. (1980). Unbiasedness of the likelihood ratio tests for equality of several covariance matrices and equality of several multivariate normal populations. *Annals of Statistics, 8*, 247-263.

Poulin, F., Dishion, T.J., & Burraston, B. (2001). Three-year iatrogenic effects associated with aggregating high-risk adolescents in cognitive-behavioral preventive interventions. *Applied Developmental Science, 5*: 214-224.

Riggs, P.D., Baker, S., Mikulich, S.K., Young, S.E., & Crowley, T.K. (1995). Depression in substance-dependent delinquents. *Journal of the American Academy of Child and Adolescent Psychiatry, 34*: 764-771.

Scheibler, D., & Schneider, W. (1985). Monte Carlo tests of the accuracy of cluster analysis algorithms–A comparison of hierarchical and nonhierarchical methods. *Multivariate Behavioral Research, 20*, 283-304.

Shaffer, D., Fisher, P., & Lucas, C. (1997). National Institute of Mental Health-Diagnostic Interview Schedule for Children-IV (NIMH-DISC IV). New York: Division of Child Psychiatry, Columbia University.

Thorndike, R. L. (1982). *Applied psychometrics.* Boston: Houghton Mifflin.

Tryon, R. C., & Bailey, D. E. (1970). *Cluster analysis.* New York: McGraw-Hill.

Ward, J. H., Jr. (1963). Hierarchical grouping to optimize an objective function. *American Statistical Association Journal, 58*, 236-244.

Weinberg, N.Z. & Glantz, M.D. (1999). Child psychopathology risk factors for drug abuse: Overview. *Journal of Clinical Child Psychology, 28*, 290-297.

Wieczorek, W.F. & Miller, B.A. (1992). Preliminary typology designed for treatment matching of driving-while-intoxicated offenders. *Journal of Consulting and Clinical Psychology, 60*, 757-765.

Winters, K.C. (1999). Treating adolescents with substance use disorders: An overview of practice issues and treatment outcomes. *Substance Abuse, 20*, 203-225.

Winters, K. C., & Stinchfield, R. D. (1995). Current issues and future needs in the assessment of adolescent drug abuse. In E. Rahdert & D. Czechowicz (Eds.), *Adolescent drug abuse: Clinical assessment and therapeutic interventions* (National Institute on Drug Abuse Research Monograph 156). Washington, DC: U.S. Government Printing Office.

doi:10.1300/J029v16n01_02

Community Readiness Survey:
Norm Development Using a Q-Sort Process

Anu Sharma
Andria M. Botzet
Rebecca A. J. Sechrist
Nikki Arthur
Ken C. Winters

SUMMARY. This study reports on norms developed for the Minnesota Institute of Public Health's (1999) Community Readiness Survey. Prevention experts from ten states and the Red Lake Nation sorted data from 50 communities into high and low readiness groups using a Q-sort process. High inter-rater agreement was achieved on communities sorted. Tests of significance between the high and low readiness groups resulted in significant differences on the five scales of readiness: community members' perception of an alcohol, tobacco, and other drug problem; permissiveness of attitudes toward substance use; support for prevention; perceived access of alcohol and tobacco products for adolescents; and overall community commitment. Communities that implement a readiness assessment can use these results to target resources to areas in which high readiness is indicated and

---

Anu Sharma and Rebecca A. J. Sechrist are affiliated with the Minnesota Institute of Public Health. Andria M. Botzet, Nikki Arthur, and Ken C. Winters are all affiliated with the Department of Psychiatry at the University of Minnesota.

Address correspondence to: Anu Sharma, Minnesota Institute of Public Health, 2720 Highway 10, Mounds View, MN 55112 (E-mail: asharma@miph.org).

[Haworth co-indexing entry note]: "Community Readiness Survey: Norm Development Using a Q-Sort Process." Sharma, Anu et al. Co-published simultaneously in *Journal of Child & Adolescent Substance Abuse* (The Haworth Press, Inc.) Vol. 16, No. 1, 2006, pp. 25-38; and: *Adolescent Substance Abuse: New Frontiers in Assessment* (ed: Ken C. Winters) The Haworth Press, Inc., 2006, pp. 25-38. Single or multiple copies of this article are available for a fee from The Haworth Document Delivery Service [1-800-HAWORTH, 9:00 a.m. - 5:00 p.m. (EST). E-mail address: docdelivery@haworthpress.com].

seek to increase readiness in areas in which lower scale scores are evidenced. doi:10.1300/J029v16n01_03 *[Article copies available for a fee from The Haworth Document Delivery Service: 1-800-HAWORTH. E-mail address: <docdelivery@haworthpress.com> Website: <http://www.HaworthPress.com> © 2006 by The Haworth Press, Inc. All rights reserved.]*

KEYWORDS. Adolescent, drug abuse, assessment

INTRODUCTION

Dryfoos (1997) estimated that 30% of 14- to 17-year-olds regularly engage in multiple high-risk behaviors, and an additional 35% experiment with various high-risk behaviors. These include, but unfortunately are not limited to, substance use, teen pregnancy, antisocial behavior, suicidal ideation and attempts, and academic failure. To address these risk behaviors, professionals have increasingly turned to family and community domains, rather than relying on interventions aimed predominantly at the individual level. "Substance abuse prevention, in the past often targeted to specific at-risk populations, has moved into an era of community oriented action in which neighborhoods rather than individuals are the target of prevention efforts" (Peyrot & Smith, 1998, p. 66).

Integral to the success of any community-oriented initiative is a systematic community-level assessment. However, as stated by Paronen and Oja (1998), "Community assessment has no defined formula" (p. S26). A major contributing factor to this is the lack of consensus regarding the term "community." Sharma (2003) notes that "community" derives from the Latin *communite,* meaning "common" or "fellowship," but "beyond acknowledging that community involves human beings, there is very little agreement on its definition" (p. 22). Hillery (1955) lists 94 definitions of community; the only common thread among these is the focus on human beings. In part, this variety exists because definitions of community can include a focus on geographic, social, or cultural elements. For purposes of community assessment, however, geographic boundaries are typically selected. Even here, though, choices arise. Hogan, Gabrielsen, Luna, and Grothaus (2003) state, for example, that a "community" can be a school, neighborhood, city block, or county.

It follows, then, that community assessment will be defined in various ways. Paronen and Oja (1998) consider assessment to be the "critical first step in planning a promotional project that takes into account and makes use of the unique characteristics of a community" (p. S26). They view it as the "process of assessing and defining needs, opportunities, and resources in a community that constitutes the basis for initiating community-based health promotion or other developmental activities" (p. S26). Inherent in this definition is a common interpretation of community-level assessment, namely, that it is largely synonymous with needs and resource assessment. However, community-level assessment is broader; it includes needs and resource assessment but should be accompanied by a parallel and equally important process–that of assessing the community's level of readiness to address risk behaviors.

The United Way of America's (1982) definition of needs assessment segues into this concept. They consider needs assessment to be ". . . a systematic process of collection and analysis as inputs into resource allocation decisions with a view to discovering and identifying goods and services the community is lacking in relation to the generally accepted standards, and *for which there exists some consensus as to the community's responsibility for their provision*" (p. 2, emphasis added). As Logan, Williams, and Leukefeld (2001) point out, the second part of this definition suggests that "merely determining a need should not be the sole consideration in resource allocation. The community must be willing to accept responsibility in meeting that need" (p. 5). The importance of community readiness, labeled here as "willingness to accept responsibility," therefore, is underscored.

Recent literature on substance abuse prevention has emphasized the importance of assessing community readiness. The Center for Substance Abuse Prevention's (CSAP) Western and Central Centers for the Application of Prevention Technologies (CAPT) (2001, 2003, respectively) list assessing community readiness as the first step in their seven-step planning process for prevention program planning. The original motivation for assessing community readiness was, in fact, presented by Pentz at the Kentucky Conference for Prevention Research in 1991. "Unless a community was ready, initiation of a prevention program was unlikely, and if a program was started despite the fact that the community was not ready, initiation was likely to lead only to failure" (Edwards, Jumper-Thurman, Plested, Oetting, & Swanson, 2000, p. 293).

In response to Pentz, over the past decade, several tools have been developed to assess community readiness. Peyrot and Smith (1998) posited and tested a model of readiness of local residents to engage in collective action to prevent substance abuse in their own neighborhood. Goodman and Wandersman (National Institute on Drug Abuse, 1997) developed a readiness survey designed for use with key leaders that assesses awareness, concern, and action across community levels. Both these tools, however, are limited in terms of their applicability. In the former case, the authors discuss the modest level of explained variance indicating that their model was not complete, as well as limitations in measurement and scoring of their instrument. In the latter case, the authors did not create a scoring mechanism for their tool; rather they recommend that potential users average item-level responses and interpret results in the context of their own community.

By far the two most utilized means of assessing Community Readiness are the Tri-Ethnic Center's (Oetting, Donnermeyer, Plested, Edwards, Kelly, & Beauvais, 1995) Community Readiness Model and the Minnesota Institute of Public Health's (MIPH) (Minnesota Institute of Public Health, 1999) Community Readiness Survey. These assessment tools are distinctly different and therefore essentially complementary. The Tri-Ethnic Center's Community Readiness Model uses key informant interviews to assess six dimensions: existing efforts, knowledge about the problem, knowledge about alternative methods or policies, leadership, resources, and community climate. Trained interviewers conduct up to 4-5 interviews per community; once results are coded, the community is categorized into one of nine stages: community tolerance/no knowledge, denial, vague awareness, preplanning, preparation, initiation, institutionalization/stabilization, confirmation/expansion, and professionalization. The model is not limited to substance abuse; rather, it can be used to assess a community's level of readiness on any number of topics. Recent examples include intimate partner violence (Brackley, Davila, Thornton, Leal, Mudd, Shafer, Castillo, & Spears, 2003), drug use (Oetting, Jumper-Thurman, Plested, & Edwards, 2001), and health services (Oetting, Jumper-Thurman, Plested, & Edwards, 2001).

The Minnesota Institute of Public Health's Community Readiness Survey utilizes a survey process with a random sample of community residents. The purpose, therefore, is that of most quantitative surveys, namely to validly estimate the proportions of community members that share a characteristic (Williams & Yanoshik, 2001). The survey is specific to alcohol, tobacco, and other drug (ATOD) use, and community residents' responses are reported on five scales: community members' perception of an ATOD problem, permissiveness of attitudes toward substance use, support for ATOD prevention, perceived access of alcohol and tobacco products for adolescents, and overall community commitment.

Psychometric development and initial validation of the MIPH Community Readiness Survey is described elsewhere (Beebe, Harrison,

Sharma, & Hedger, 2001). However, this previous study, which demonstrated internal validity of the five scales, was limited by the lack of development of norms for these scales. The value in providing normative data is clear; norms provide a context for communities in which to interpret their own results. Given such a context, communities would be more able to target resources to areas in which high readiness is indicated and seek to increase readiness where needed. The purpose of this study is to provide norms for scales on the MIPH Community Readiness Survey, thereby enhancing its applicability for communities.

METHODS

Sample

Fifty communities located primarily in the upper Midwest region of the United States comprised the sample for this study. Thirty were from the original validation study conducted by Beebe et al. (2001), and 20 communities were included that had implemented the survey since that time. The original validation study included 50 communities; however, the decision not to include all 50 was based on using as little as possible the same sample on which the scales were originally developed and internally validated. Ideally, when faced with the task of norming, one wishes to have as large a sample as possible; however, because the unit of analysis is community versus individual respondent, the resources required prohibit the gathering of a large sample. Fifty communities, therefore, was considered an adequate minimum on which to norm.

The total number of participants in the 50 communities numbered 10,728, which represented an overall response rate of 44%. In terms of gender, 52.3% of the sample was male, indicating an overall gender balance. The Community Readiness Survey is designed for adults 18 and older; hence all respondents were in this age range. Highest levels of respondents tended to occur in the 35- to 44-year-old and 65 and older age categories; approximately half the sample fell into these two age groups. Ethnic minorities comprised 10.7% of the sample.

Measures

The measures and procedures used for the sample of 30 communities from the original validation study is described in Beebe et al. (2001). Samples of 500 were randomly drawn in each of these communities, and the Dillman (1978) method was utilized to maximize response rates.

In the 20 subsequent communities, surveys were sent to 600 randomly selected respondents in each community. (This sample size was chosen because it allows for a 7% or less margin of error on each item.) Each community level sample consisted of a random sample of directory-listed household addresses purchased from Survey Sampling, Inc., of Westport, Connecticut. Three mailings were sent to each household address: (1) prenotification letter announcing the survey, sent one week in advance of the survey, (2) survey with self-addressed, stamped envelope, and (3) reminder postcard sent one week later. Two methods were employed to boost response rates. First, the prenotification letter was signed by a local leader and written on local letterhead, usually representing the agency or organization sponsoring the survey. Second, a small incentive was included with the survey. These were chosen individually by community; examples included pens, refrigerator magnets, coupons to local businesses, etc.

Respondents were asked to complete the survey and mail it anonymously in the self-addressed, stamped envelope. The survey consists of 52 items, 46 of which fall into one of the five scales, with an additional 6 being demographic in nature. Scales, sample items, and scale score interpretations are shown in Table 1.

TABLE 1. Community Readiness Survey Scales

Scale	Descriptor	Score Interpretation
Perception of ATOD problem	To what extent do residents believe ATOD use is a problem in their community?	Higher score = more perception Lower score = less perception
Permissiveness of attitudes toward ATOD use	To what extent do community members view ATOD use as "okay" or "no big deal"?	Higher score = more permissive Lower score = less permissive
Support for ATOD prevention	How much support would community members give to ATOD prevention?	Higher score = more support Lower score = less support
Perceived adolescent access to alcohol and tobacco	How easy do residents think it is for adolescents to obtain alcohol and tobacco in their community?	Higher score = more access Lower score = less access
Community commitment	Is this community apathetic in general?	Higher score = more apathy Lower score = less apathy

Procedure

After data had been received from the 50 communities, percentages were calculated for each of the response options by community. In many cases, two response options were combined to indicate percent agreement with a given item. For example, in response to the item, "In my community, drinking among teenagers is acceptable," the percentages of respondents who endorsed "Strongly agree" or "Agree" were combined and reported as a single percentage indicative of overall agreement with this item.

Using these percentages, five data sheets were created for each community, one for each scale. Each data sheet reported on the percentage of respondents who endorsed items on that scale, with each item reported individually. These data sheets were then organized by scale and ranked by prevention experts utilizing a Q-sort technique.

The Q-sort, developed originally by Stephenson (1953), is a method that facilitates prioritization or ranking of complex data in a relatively timely fashion. A central characteristic of this process is that it is a comparative rather than absolute rating method. Raters are asked to sort stimuli in terms of a fixed distribution, and in preparation to the actual sorting, are instructed to place the stimuli into three gross classes–two at each extreme of the distribution and a third, those about which the rater is ambivalent. That is, the rater is instructed to work from both ends of the continuum toward the middle. The rationale for this is that extremes tend to be more quickly discerned than less extreme cases. The end result is that cases are sorted into a fixed distribution. According to Nunnally (1967), "the major reason for using the Q-sort rather than some other comparative rating method is that it greatly conserves the time taken to make ratings" (p. 546).

In the case of the Community Readiness Survey, 20 raters were trained to independently sort data from the 50 communities using the data sheets provided. These raters were prevention experts associated with CSAP's Central CAPT and had been brought together in August 2001 to Minneapolis, MN as part of their ongoing professional development. These Associates are housed in ten states (Ohio, West Virginia, Illinois, Indiana, Michigan, Wisconsin, Minnesota, Iowa, North Dakota, South Dakota) and the Red Lake Nation. They represent a variety of sectors (state agencies, schools, community-based organizations, public health, faith community, etc.) and were selected as CSAP's Central CAPT Associates based on a competitive process, a key element of which was experience and knowledge about prevention within their states. Hence, they were deemed as possessing expert knowledge appropriate for the Community Readiness Survey Q-sort task.

In accordance with standard Q-sort instructions, these experts examined the data sheets that contained percent endorsement of scale items and placed communities with data representing high readiness in one pile and communities representing low readiness in a second pile. Ambiguous data were placed in a third pile by each rater and then force sorted into either high or low readiness. The end result was to ensure that both piles had an equal number of communities (i.e., 25 high readiness and 25 low readiness).

Scales 1 through 4 were each sorted by five different raters, and Scale 5 was rated by 19 sorters (one of the 20 sorters left the sorting process early due to a family emergency). Thus, all 19 raters sorted Scale 5 plus one other scale.

Analysis

Two primary data analyses were conducted. First, ratings were compared across sorters to determine the percent of rater agreement. Second, calculations were made on the high and low readiness groups in an effort to establish scale norms. Mean scores and standard deviations were computed at the item and scale level for communities in the high and low readiness groups. T-tests and Mann-Whitney (nonparametric) tests of significance were conducted on the difference in mean scores between the two groups.

RESULTS

Rater Agreement

Figure 1 shows the rater agreement on each of the five scales. Percent agreement was highest for Scales 1 and 5. On Scale 1, 72% of the communities were sorted by the 5 raters exactly the same way (i.e., high and low readiness piles) and on Scale 5, 76% of the communities were sorted by all 19 raters into the same high and low readiness piles. On the other three scales, there was also considerable agreement across raters. On Scales 2, 3, and 4, 62%, 70%, and 82%, respectively, had either complete agreement on communities sorted or had only one rater who disagreed with the sorting process of the other raters. (For example, on Scale 2, 48% of the communities were sorted exactly the same by all

FIGURE 1. Rater agreement (5 raters for each of Scales 1, 2, and 3; 4 raters for Scale 4; and 19 raters for Scale 5)

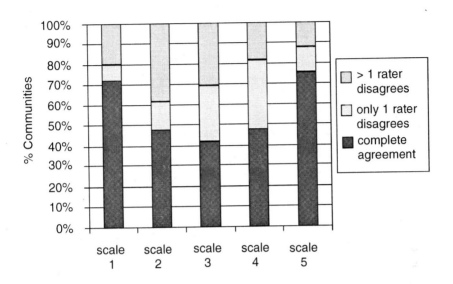

five raters, and an additional 14% of the communities had one rater who did not sort exactly the same as the other four raters.) Overall, it appears that there was considerable consensus across raters regarding which communities were characterized as being high and low readiness.

Scale Norms

Table 2 shows the results of t-tests of significance conducted on the differences between mean scale scores of the high and low readiness community groups. Also displayed are nonparametric Mann-Whitney test statistics and corresponding p-values. On all five scales, significant differences were found between the high and low readiness groups on both the parametric and nonparametric tests.

Similar tests of significance (t-tests and Mann-Whitney tests) were conducted at the item level. That is, all survey items were tested to detect significant mean differences between the high and low readiness groups. With the exception of four items, the two groups were significantly different at the .05 or lower level of significance. On 36 items, the two groups were significantly different at the $p < .0001$ level.

TABLE 2. Tests of Significance on Mean Scale Scores for High and Low Readiness Communities

Scale	T-Statistic	p-value	Mann-Whitney	p-value
Perception of ATOD problem	−16.8	.000	−11.7	.000
Permissiveness of attitudes toward ATOD use	−10.1	.000	−9.8	.000
Support for ATOD prevention	−11.5	.000	−9.5	.000
Perceived adolescent access to alcohol and tobacco	−8.5	.000	−7.7	.000
Community commitment	−39.0	.000	−26.2	.000

The four exceptions occurred on Scale 2 ("In my community, drinking among teenagers is acceptable"), Scale 3 ("To help pay for prevention service, how willing would you be to increase taxes on tobacco?") and Scale 4 ("How difficult is it for teenagers in your community to sneak alcohol from their home or a friend's home?" and "How difficult is it for teenagers in your community to sneak tobacco products from their home or a friend's home?"). The items from Scales 2 and 4 showed "wrong directionality," that is, the mean item scores were higher for the low readiness communities than for the high readiness communities. The item from Scale 3, while the means were in the "right direction," resulted in no significant difference between the two groups. These findings indicate that at an item level, for nearly all the items, discrimination occurred between the low and high readiness groups.

DISCUSSION

Based on these results, it appears that norms were successfully developed to better define high and low readiness communities. The Q-sort process resulted in sufficiently high inter-rater agreement on communities sorted into low and high readiness groups. Subsequent analyses and significance tests on mean differences between these groups showed significant differences on all five community readiness scales and nearly all survey items.

The implication of these findings is clear: Communities that elect to administer the MIPH Community Readiness Survey have a context in which to interpret their findings. Comparisons can be made between specific community data obtained and norms representing high and low readiness community groups. On a practical level, communities would then be better able to target resources. For example, a community in which residents do not perceive adolescent substance use as problematic (low readiness on the perception scale) can be dealt with differently than a community in which the problem has been identified but residents are unsure as to what actions are required. Another example is one in which low readiness is indicated on community commitment scale. In this case, community leaders and prevention professionals may need to place substance abuse prevention within the context of issues that community members identify as more pressing, e.g., unemployment, housing, economic development. In general, community leaders, prevention professionals, and residents can seek to capitalize on areas in which the community demonstrates high readiness, while increasing readiness in areas in which lower scale scores are reported.

Several cautions, however, should be noted. Communities should use these norms as context only, as opposed to a "gold standard" for which to aim. That is, the mean and/or range of the high readiness communities is a relative rather than an absolute standard. Community residents and leaders should still seek to determine acceptable and/or optimal goals for their own communities on each of the five dimensions.

This has special relevance for ethnically diverse communities. As noted in the methods section, the 50 communities on which the norming process occurred were predominantly upper Midwestern communities primarily populated by Caucasians. Plested, Smitham, Jumper-Thurman, Oetting, and Edwards (1999), in a study of 102 rural Caucasian and minority communities, found that while most rural communities were at relatively low stages of readiness, minority rural communities were even lower. Only 2% of the minority communities had functioning drug prevention programs, in contrast to 30% of the White American communities assessed as being at the initiation stage of readiness or above. The authors concluded that "major efforts aimed at providing prevention programs in rural communities are needed, particularly in minority communities" (p. 536).

The norms developed in this study, therefore, may not be applicable to ethnically diverse communities. As additional community data are gathered, particularly on ethnically diverse communities, appropriate norms may need to be developed for different subpopulations.

Another limitation of this study is that the norming process was conducted by experts, rather than by sampling standardization groups. This was due primarily to the unit of analysis being community rather than individual, which in turn, severely limited the sample size. As additional communities implement the Community Readiness Survey, it may be useful to repeat the norming process with another group of experts and an additional sample of communities. This, too, would help eliminate the bias that may have arisen from 30 of the communities having also been part of the original validation study conducted by Beebe et al. (2001).

Despite these limitations, however, the results obtained through this norming process are encouraging and increase the potential that communities will more broadly utilize readiness assessments. Locally based data, such as obtained through a community-level readiness survey, is likely to prove invaluable. "National or regional data are likely to be viewed as meaningless since every rural community, with some justification, sees itself as unique, so local survey data may be valuable in moving the community toward action" (Plested, Smitham, Jumper-Thurman, Oetting, & Edwards, 1999, p. 531). This is the case not only with rural communities but other communities as well. "Efforts by *local* people are likely to have the greatest and most sustainable impact in solving *local* problems and in setting *local* norms . . . Successful prevention programs are 'owned' by the targeted community itself" (emphasis in original, Edwards et al., 2000, p. 292). And, as echoed by Mills and Bogenschneider (2001), "local citizens can assess the extent of community risk for adolescent alcohol use . . . contradict[ing] naysayers who question the ability of local citizens to reliably assess such support" (p. 365).

No doubt that community readiness is a field yet in its infancy. However, "identification of the starting point is key to the eventual success and sustainability of any prevention program" (Edwards et al., 2000, p. 293). The ultimate goal is to increase the likelihood that adolescent substance use prevention programs will succeed, thereby decreasing the rates of adolescent substance use and related risk behaviors. If multi-sector and community-based initiatives are to contribute to this process, then community readiness has a role. "Knowing the community and its constituents is more than an epidemiological assessment" (Nicola & Hatcher, 2000, p. 4.) It is, in fact, more than a needs or resource assessment. Operating from a base that includes knowledge of community members' readiness to address adolescent substance use will give a decided advantage to those concerned with reducing adolescent risk behaviors.

REFERENCES

Beebe, T., J., Harrison, P. A., Sharma, A., & Hedger, S. (2001). The Community Readiness Survey: Development and initial validation. *Evaluation Review, 25,* 55-71.

Brackley, M., Davila, Y., Thornton, J., Leal, C., Mudd, G., Shafer, J., Castillo, P., & Spears, W. (2003). Community readiness to prevent intimate partner violence in Bexar County, Texas. *Journal of Transcultural Nursing, 14,* 227-236.

Center for Substance Abuse Prevention's (CSAP) Central Center for the Application of Prevention Technologies (CAPT). (2003). *Substance Abuse Prevention Specialist Training.* Mounds View, MN: CSAP's Central CAPT.

Center for Substance Abuse Prevention's (CSAP) Western Center for the Application of Prevention Technologies (CAPT). (2001). *Substance Abuse Prevention Specialist Training.* Reno, NV: CSAP's Western CAPT.

Dryfoos, J. G. (1997). The prevalence of problem behaviors: Implications for programs. In R.P. Weissberg, T. P. Gullotta, R. L. Hampton, & G. R. Adams (Eds.), *Healthy children 2010: Enhancing children's wellness* (pp. 17-46). Newbury Park, CA: Sage.

Edwards, R. W., Jumper-Thurman, P., Plested, B. A., Oetting, E. R., & Swanson, L. (2000). Community readiness: Research to practice. *Journal of Community Psychology, 28,* 291-307.

Hillery, G. A. (1955). Definitions of community: Areas of agreement. *Rural Sociology, 20,* 111-125.

Hogan, J. A., Gabrielsen, K. R., Luna, N., & Grothaus, D. (2003). *Substance abuse prevention: The intersection of science and practice.* Boston: Pearson Education.

Logan, T. K., Williams, K., & Leukefeld, C. (2001). A statewide drug court needs assessment: Identifying target counties, assessing readiness. *Journal of Offender Rehabilitation, 33,* 1-25.

Mills, J., & Bogenschneider, K. (2001). Can communities assess support for preventing adolescent alcohol and other drug use? Reliability and validity of a community assessment inventory. *Family Relations, 50,* 355-375.

Minnesota Institute of Public Health. (1999). *MIPH Community Readiness Survey* [survey instrument]. Mounds View, MN: Minnesota Institute of Public Health.

National Institute on Drug Abuse. (1997). *Community readiness for drug abuse prevention: Issues, tips, and tools.* Rockville, MD: U. S. Department of Health and Human Services.

Nicola, R. M., & Hatcher, M. T. (2000). A framework for building effective public health constituencies. *Journal of Public Health Management Practice, 6,* 1-10.

Nunnally, J. C. (1967). *Psychometric theory.* New York: McGraw Hill.

Oetting, E. R., Donnermeyer, J. F., Plested, B. A., Edwards, R. W., Kelly, K., & Beauvais, F. (1995). Assessing community readiness for prevention. *The International Journal of the Addictions, 30,* 659-683.

Oetting, E. R., Jumper-Thurman, P., Plested, B., & Edwards, R. W. (2001). Community readiness and health services. *Substance Use & Misuse, 36,* 825-843.

Paronen, O., & Oja, P. (1998). How to understand a community–Community assessment for the promotion of health-related physical activity. *Patient Education and Counseling, 33,* S25-S28.

Peyrot, M. & Smith, H. L. (1998). Community readiness for substance abuse prevention: Toward a model of collective action. *Research in Community Sociology, 8,* 65-91.

Plested, B., Smitham, D., M., Jumper-Thurman, P., Oetting, E. R., & Edwards, R. W. (1999). Readiness for drug use prevention in rural minority communities. *Substance Use & Misuse, 34,* 521-544.

Sharma, R. K. (2003). Putting the community back in community health assessment: A process and outcome approach with a review of some major issues for public health professionals. *Journal of Health & Social Policy, 16,* 19-33.

Stephenson, W. (1953). *The study of behavior.* Chicago: University of Chicago Press.

United Way of America. (1982). *Needs assessment: The state of the art.* Alexandria, VA.

Williams, R. L., & Yanoshik, K. (2001). Can you do a community assessment without talking to the community? *Journal of Community Health, 26,* 233-247.

doi:10.1300/J029v16n01_03

Screening American Indian Youth for Referral to Drug Abuse Prevention and Intervention Services

Ken C. Winters
Jerome DeWolfe
Donald Graham
Wehnona St. Cyr

SUMMARY. The development and psychometric properties of a brief screening tool for use with American Indian youth suspected of abusing substances is described. The Indian Health Service-Personal Experience Screening Questionnaire (IHS-PESQ) is a brief questionnaire that screens for drug abuse problem severity, response distortion tendencies, and psychosocial risk factors. The psychometric properties of the problem severity scale are favorable when tested in reservation-based American

Ken C. Winters, PhD, is affiliated with Department of Psychiatry, University of Minnesota. Jerome DeWolfe, MS, and Donald Graham are affiliated with Aberdeen Area Indian Health Service, and Wehnona St. Cyr is affiliated with Carl T. Curtis Health Center, Omaha Tribe of Nebraska.

Address correspondence to Ken C. Winters, PhD, Department of Psychiatry, University of Minnesota, F282/2A West, 2450 Riverside Avenue, Minneapolis, MN 55454.

The authors wish to express their gratitude to the numerous school officials and students who supported the collection of the surveys.

Support for this study was provided by funds from the Aberdeen Area Indian Health Service and by grants from NIDA (DA05104) and The Saint Paul Foundation to Ken C. Winters.

[Haworth co-indexing entry note]: "Screening American Indian Youth for Referral to Drug Abuse Prevention and Intervention Services." Winters, Ken C. et al. Co-published simultaneously in *Journal of Child & Adolescent Substance Abuse* (The Haworth Press, Inc.) Vol. 16, No. 1, 2006, pp. 39-52; and: *Adolescent Substance Abuse: New Frontiers in Assessment* (ed: Ken C. Winters) The Haworth Press, Inc., 2006, pp. 39-52. Single or multiple copies of this article are available for a fee from The Haworth Document Delivery Service [1-800-HAWORTH, 9:00 a.m. - 5:00 p.m. (EST). E-mail address: docdelivery@haworthpress.com].

Indian students (grades 6-12). The paper also describes the role of the IHS-PESQ within a prevention, intervention and treatment referral system designed for American Indian youth. doi:10.1300/J029v16n01_04

[Article copies available for a fee from The Haworth Document Delivery Service: 1-800-HAWORTH. E-mail address: <docdelivery@haworthpress.com> Website: <http://www.HaworthPress.com> © 2006 by The Haworth Press, Inc. All rights reserved.]

KEYWORDS. Adolescent, drug abuse, assessment

There have been several meaningful advances in the adolescent drug abuse research treatment field since the early 1990s (Weinberg, Rahdert, Colliver & Glantz, 1998; Williams & Chang, 2000). Controlled clinical trials based on empirical-driven family treatment models have been reported in the literature indicating treatment efficacy for adolescent drug abusers and descriptive studies have supported the effectiveness of Twelve-Step and cognitive-behavioral approaches as well (Winters, 1999).

However, the current health service delivery system for adolescent drug abusers is dominated by intensive services targeted for the severe-end cases that have advanced to a substance dependence disorder (CSAT, 1999). Youth with a substance abuse disorder or subclinical manifestations of drug involvement typically lack referral options in the current cost-conscious treatment environment. Most community-based treatment systems allocate their limited resources to the most severe cases and few, if any, treatment options are available for youth with less severe problem density. Thus, one area of under-development in the adolescent treatment field is intervention for adolescents with mild and moderate problems related to alcohol and other drug (AOD) involvement.

This state of treatment services suggests that there is a need for a wider spectrum of interventions than is routinely available. The implication is that the specialized treatment sector that focuses on individuals with substantial to severe AOD problems cannot be the sole focus of treatment options. If significant inroads are to be made into the overall problem of adolescent drug abuse, a broad-based therapeutic approach must be taken in which gradations of therapeutic services are tailored to meet the needs of adolescents with varying degrees of drug problems (Rahdert, 1991).

The Aberdeen Area Indian Health Service, Division of Field Health, has developed a program in order to address this service delivery gap for Indian adolescents suspected of drug involvement, the Aberdeen Area Adolescent Alcohol and Other Drug Abuse Prevention System (AODAPS). AODAPS was intended to address two needs. One need is related to the high rate of drug problems among Indian youth living in the region served by the Aberdeen Area Indian Health Service. There is no national comprehensive database of Indian youth drug use (Moran & Reaman, 2002), yet several local and regional studies have been conducted. These investigators provide evidence that use of alcohol and other drugs by Indian youth is widely variable across gender and age groups and in many instances, use is higher among Indian youth than non-Indians (Beauvais, 1992; Mail & Johnson, 1993; Walker et al., 1996). Consistent with these studies in the literature, surveys of youth in two tribal communities in the Aberdeen Area also indicate high rates of drug involvement among students (Winters & Botzet, 2002). Rates in 2002 of AOD problems when assessed with a screening measure ranged from 6%-18% among sixth graders to 50%-56% among high school seniors across schools. The second need addressed by AODAPS is aimed at correcting a major service delivery gap in the region. There is no systematic and coordinated program of identification, referral and treatment for drug-abusing American Indian youth in the Aberdeen Area.

AODAPs' core component is organized around a model of intervention and treatment services continuum described by the Institute of Medicine (IOM) in their book, *Broadening the Base of Treatment for Alcohol Problems* (IOM, 1990). As portrayed in Figure 1, the model posits that the percentage of individuals in various problem groups varies as a function of problem severity. Thus, the smallest proportion of youth in any given community is expected to be those with severe AOD problems and for whom intensive and specialized services are appropriate, whereas a largest number of youth are believed to be those who have few or any drug problems. An intermediate group, that is, those with mild to moderate problems, is believed to represent a middle-range number of youth in a given community. Brief interventions are expected to benefit these individuals.

The Aberdeen Area officials observed that implementation of the IOM model would require a reliable and valid assessment instrument to assist in identifying groups of youth that varied in problem severity and for whom varying intensities of intervention and treatment would be appropriate. A review of the assessment literature was undertaken to iden-

FIGURE 1. Aberdeen Area Alcohol and Other Drug Prevention System

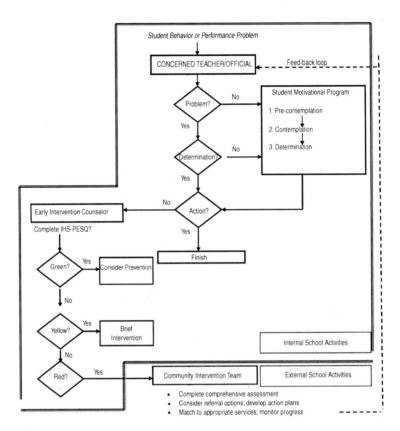

tify a psychometrically sound instrument to serve as an initial screening tool for use in an IOM-adapted model. Specifically, the candidate instrument had to be associated with validity evidence as a measure of drug abuse problem severity, and show potential as a valid instrument to assist with intervention and treatment referral decisions.

The Personal Experience Screening Questionnaire (PESQ) (Winters, 1992) was selected for consideration in AODAPS. The PESQ showed potential to meet the program goals in that it produced a continuous problem severity score with substantial variance when administered to heterogeneous populations of drug-using teenagers, and it contained empirically-validated cut scores to distinguish AOD problem severity groups. However, because the PESQ had only one cut point to distinguish two groups (no or minimal AOD problem versus AOD problem), more validation was needed in order to determine the instrument's potential to identify the three problem severity groups as specified by AODAPS (no AOD problem versus mild or moderate AOD problem versus severe AOD problem).

The present study focuses on the use of the PESQ within the AODAPs. Specifically, we evaluated the psychometric properties of the PESQ when used in a youth Indian population, including the instrument's validity as a measure of distinct problem severity groups. Also, the potential utility of the PESQ for problem identification in a multiple-gating referral system is discussed.

INITIAL SCALE DEVELOPMENT
AND PSYCHOMETRICS OF THE PESQ

Subjects. Subjects that participated in the study to develop the original PESQ have been described previously (Winters, 1992). Briefly, participants ranged in age from 12 to 18 years and were receiving drug abuse evaluation at 16 Minnesota drug clinic assessment programs (either residential or outpatient). The 646 participants were male, between the ages of 15 and 17, 89% was White, and all were tested prior to treatment. The sample was divided into two groups: a *development* sample (n = 398) which was used to identify the new screening items, and a *replication* sample (n = 248) for use in preliminary reliability and validity evaluations. The samples were defined by splitting the subjects at approximately the calendar halfway point of data collection procedures. A comparison was made between participants and nonparticipants in the development sample. Between-group analyses (participants vs. nonparticipants) failed to detect statistically significant differences on demographic characteristics (sex, age, race, prior treatment history), psychological variables (MMPI validity and clinical scales), and total drug use frequency. Also, comparisons were made between participants in the development and replication samples on these same variables; between-group analyses (development vs. replication) failed to detect any statistically significant differences.

Procedure. The first criteria for selection as a screening item was membership in a problem severity general factor identified in previous assessment research (see Henly & Winters, 1988). The factor was identified from a principal component factor analysis based on responses by the development sample to 136 problem severity items representing seven relevant drug abuse content areas. These a priori content areas and their items had been rationally identified based on empirical findings from adolescent and adult problem severity studies and on service provider opinions about the nature of adolescent AOD abuse. Scale-based items were formatted to have two (yes/no), three (never/once or twice/more than once or twice), or four (never/once or twice/sometimes/often) response options; the AOD use frequency items were formatted on a 7-point scale (1 = never; 7 = 40 +).

A principal component factor analysis using polychoric correlations was applied to the 136 problem severity items. A general factor, consisting of 66 items with loadings ≥ .50, was identified. Twenty-nine items were assigned to a larger questionnaire, the Personal Experience Inventory (PEI) (Winters & Henly, 1988). The remaining 37 general factor items not assigned to this PEI scale were viewed as an item pool from which the screening scale could be developed. Eighteen items were identified as desirable because each were formatted with a 4-point response option scheme (never/once or twice/sometimes/often). A consistent item format was viewed as desirable because it simplifies hand scoring procedures. Each selected item was scaled in the same direction such that endorsement reflected drug use problem severity.

A principal component factor analysis was performed on the 18-item set. Only one factor was identified (eigenvalue of 6.8; percent of variance, 38.1). Item factor loadings ranged from .50 to .74 (median, .62). Separate principal component factor analyses also were computed for males and females. In each analysis, a single factor was identified with similar eiginvalues (7.0 for males and 6.8 for females), percents of variance (39.0 for males and 38.0 for females), and item factor loadings (range for males, .50 to .77; range for females, .52 to .73).

Finally, these additional items of clinical relevance were added to the 18-item problem severity set to form the full PESQ: (a) several drug use frequency (DUF) items (past 12 months) that were adapted from Johnston, Backman, and O'Malley (1986); (b) five items (Defensiveness) adapted from the Marlowe-Crowne Social Desirability scale, a commonly used measure of defensive response tendencies (Crowne & Marlowe, 1969); (c) three items (Infrequency) that address highly improbable events (e.g., buying drugs from a security guard); and five psychosocial risk items (e.g, suicidal tendency). Item wording reflected a sixth-grade reading level (Fry, 1977).

Original psychometrics. Several psychometric analyses were conducted on the 18-item problem severity scale using the adjusted replication drug clinic sample (n = 227) from the 1984 study and three new samples (normal school, juvenile offender, and school clinic) collected between 1987 and 1988. The normal school and juvenile offender groups were collected to examine internal consistency for new samples and to provide relevant discriminant validity tests. The school clinic group was specifically collected to evaluate the scale's criterion validity (predicting need for comprehensive assessment referral). As reported elsewhere (Winters, 1992), favorable internal consistency (coefficient alpha) data across all gender, age and setting groups were obtained, and favorable discriminant validity data (school vs. juvenile offender and school vs. drug clinic) were obtained as well.

REVISING AND VALIDATING THE PESQ FOR USE IN AODAPS

Based on consultation with Aberdeen Area officials, two revisions to the PESQ were made in order to better accommodate its use with native youth. First, Peyote and Mescaline was dropped from the list of hallucinogens given their possible use as medicine in native religious ceremonies. Second, the scoring rules of the 18-item problem severity scale were revised so that three mutually exclusive groups could be identified: no AOD problem (green flag), mild/moderate AOD problem (yellow flag), and severe AOD problem (red flag). The original PESQ problem severity scale had a single cut score to identify youth into one of two groups, either "green flag" (no problem) or "red flag" (problem). The two-group distinction, however, does not readily identify an intermediate group of youth that display mild or moderate drug involvement. This intermediate group is of great interest to the AODAPS model given that both problem severity and intervention response are viewed along a continuum. In this light, the model conceptualized mild-to-moderate cases as needing a brief intervention. Accordingly, officials at the Aberdeen Area Indian Health Service rationally identified new cut points in order that three flag groups would be identified. The new cut scores produced the same cut score for the original red flag group but produced a much narrower score range for the original green flag group. That is, the additional cut score was placed at roughly the mid-point of the original score range for the green flag group.

The revised PESQ (referred to here to as the IHS-PESQ) was then empirically tested on an existing database previously used to validate the original PESQ (Winters, 1991). This data set consists of junior and senior high school students who were referred to school chemical health counselors for an evaluation based on an in-school drug use incident.

Counselors, who were blind to PESQ scores, rated whether the student needed an evaluation for a full assessment. Given that the data also included a counselor rating as to whether the student would benefit from one of three service options (no services needed vs. low intensive treatment vs. intensive treatment), we were in a position to examine the accuracy of the revised cut scores on a validation sample. The analysis revealed that the IHS-PESQ yielded cut scores that correctly classified 91% of the students by service option.

METHOD

Subjects. Students in grades 6-12 at several Midwestern tribal-based schools were administered the IHS-PESQ during one of either of two school years (1999-2000 or 2000-2001). Administration was conducted in a classroom setting, participation was voluntary, and students were promised confidentiality and anonymity. The sample characteristics are summarized in Table 1.

Procedure. The procedures for administering the IHS-PESQ were equivalent to those used when the original PESQ was administered to school samples: students were assured of anonymity and confidentiality of results; participation was voluntary; testing occurred in a group setting. The senior author monitored all testing sessions.

RESULTS

Prior to the data analysis, cases were omitted if (a) more than 10% of the items were unscorable, or if either of the validity scales (Defensive-

TABLE 1. Sample Sizes and IHS-PESQ Flag Status of the Student Groups (grades 6 through 12) Tested at the Aberdeen Area Indian Health Service School Sites (1999 to 2001)

Group	n (%)	Green Flag %	Yellow Flag %	Red Flag %
Total	985	57	22	21
Boys	517 (53)	60	19	21
Girls	468 (48)	53	26	21
Grades 6-8	589 (60)	66	20	14
Grades 9-12	396 (40)	43	26	31

ness and Infrequency) were elevated. These rules led to the exclusion of 7% of cases.

Reliability

Internal consistency (coefficient alpha) reliability data of the problem severity scale are reported in Table 2. Any scale with a coefficient alpha above .70 is considered favorable, and above .90 is considered very favorable (Nunnally, 1967). The data indicate that estimates of the scale's internal consistency reliability are either favorable or very favorable for all groups defined by sex and grade. No coefficient alpha was below .81 and many alphas exceeded .90.

Convergent Validity

Drug use frequency. The first analysis examined recent (prior 12 months) DUF as a function of flag group (green, yellow, red). Summing (nonweighted) the three DUF items created a composite variable (range 3-21). We computed separate one-way (flag group) ANOVAs for each grade on this composite drug use frequency variable. It was predicted that the three flag groups would differ significantly on drug use and that group means will be rank-ordered as expected (green flag < yellow flag < red flag). The results provide confirming evidence that flag groups differed significantly on the DUF. All ANOVAs were significant at the $p <$ .01 level. Also, all post-hoc pairwise comparisons showed a pattern of DUF scores as expected (green flag < yellow flag < red flag), and except for grades 6 and 7, all pairwise tests (Student-Newman-Keuls) were significant ($p < .05$). A related analysis examined the magnitude of the relationship between the continuous score on the problem severity scale and the composite DUF. These results were consistent with the categor-

TABLE 2. Internal Consistency Reliability on the IHS-PESQ Problem Severity Scale by Gender and Grade Groups

Group	α
Total	.92
Boys	.93
Girls	.92
Grades 6-8	.90
Grades 9-12	.91

ical analysis: The IHS-PESQ scale was highly correlated with DUF (see Table 3). All correlations were statistically significant ($p < .01$; range .77-82). The magnitude of these correlations indicates that the problem severity scale reflects, to a large degree, the same construct measured by the DUF variable.

Psychosocial risk factors. Next we examined the association between the number of psychosocial risks and flag group membership. The psychosocial risk score was based on the number of endorsements on the IHS-PESQ risk items (range 0-5). It is predicted that flag group status would be associated with psychosocial risk status in the expected direction. Table 4 summarizes the estimate of risk for yellow flag or red flag status based on the count of psychosocial factors using the odds ratio (OR) statistic. The OR statistic will indicate the increased likelihood of being either yellow or red flag, as opposed to green flag status, as a function of the number of psychosocial risks. An OR of 1.0 means there is no increased likelihood of yellow/red flag status compared to green flag status in the presence of the respective number of psychosocial risks, and ORs significantly greater than 1.0 or less than 1.0 reflect whether there is an increase or decrease in likelihood of yellow/red flag status given the number of psychosocial risks present. The pattern of results indicate that the presence of 3 or 4 risk factors significantly increases the likelihood of a yellow/red flag status in all subject groups, and having no risk factors significantly decreases such a likelihood in all subject groups.

Factor Structure

The unidimensionality of the problem severity scale was evaluated. A principal component analysis indicated that the scale was represented by one factor for all groups (eigenvalues = 6.9-8.0), accounting for 38%

TABLE 3. Pearson Product-Moment Correlation of the IHS-PESQ Problem Severity Scale and Drug Composite Use Frequency Variable by Gender and Grade Groups

Group	r
Total	.82
Boys	.82
Girls	.82
Grades 6-8	.77
Grades 9-12	.81

Note: all correlation coefficients are significant at the $p < .001$ level.

TABLE 4. Extent to Which (Odds Ratio) the Number of Risk Factors (0-4) Increases the Likelihood of Yellow or Red Flag Status

Group	0 risks	1 risk	2 risks	3 risks	4 risks
Total	.45*	.87	1.35	2.94*	2.91*
Boys	.57*	.90	1.47	2.11*	3.09*
Girls	.30*	.83	1.26	3.90*	2.81*
Grades 6-8	.34*	.55*	1.78	5.25*	4.73*
Grades 9-12	.39*	1.32	1.50	2.60*	2.89*

[1] The odds ratio statistic was not computed for the group with 5 risks because of too many empty cells across most groups.

* $p < .01$

(grades 6-8) to 45% (boys) of the variance. In only one group (grades 6-8) was a second factor with an eigenvalue over 1.00 identified; this factor accounted for only 7% of the variance.

DISCUSSION

While limited to self-report data, the study generally supports the utility of the IHS-PESQ for use in screening American Indian youth for drug involvement. First, we consistently obtained favorable internal consistency reliability coefficients across all gender and age groups. Coefficient alphas were in excess of .88 for all subgroups. These favorable internal consistency data support the view that the problem severity items of the screen were drawn from a relevant item pool reflecting drug abuse experiences of Indian youth. The principal component analysis provides support that the scale is undimensional in all groups.

A second major finding is that the convergent validity data revealed predictably higher coefficients of the problem severity scale with the aggregate drug use frequency scale compared with the aggregate psychosocial scale. However, it is not unexpected that we found a significant association between the problem severity and psychosocial scales given the wealth of adolescent research on the strong link between drug use and psychosocial risk factors (Kaminer, 1994), including among native youth populations (Walker et al., 1996).

The third major conclusion from the data indicates that, generally speaking, response distortion elevations ("faking bad" and "faking good") were consistently low across the subgroups (range, 4%-8%). Moreover, the number of invalid cases due to excessive unscorable responses (i.e., more than 20% of the items on the test are unscorable due to either no response marked or multiple responses are marked) was less than 0.4%. Both of these sets of response distortion data suggest that the IHS-PESQ does not yield prohibitively high rates of invalid protocols when used with American youth.

A final conclusion from the data is that the psychometric data obtained on the 18-item problem severity scale when administered to American Indian youth were comparable to psychometric evidence obtained in prior studies when the same 18-item scale was used tested with samples that were primarily white (Winters, 1992). We conducted a post-hoc analysis of the reliability and validity data between American Indian and white samples and found that comparable subgroups based on age and gender did not differ. Likewise, the rates of response distortion tendencies did not differ between the two groups. These findings of psychometric comparability across ethnic groups provide initial support that use of the IHS-PESQ in American Indian youth does not lead to poorer psychometric properties compared to the use of the original PESQ when used in largely white samples.

There are study limitations to consider when interpreting the findings. We had some, but minor, nonparticipation at the various testing sessions due to absenteeism. Based on the best available data, absenteeism was typically below 5% for any given testing date. Also, the criterion measures were imperfect and of limited scope. Given that these measures were also based on youth self-report, our validity coefficients benefited from shared method variance. Also, the present study is incomplete in light of the fact that ultimately, the predictive validity of the IHS-PESQ needs to be evaluated in the context of its incremental value in matching drug abuse severity with response intensity. For example, it will be important to empirically test whether mild-to-moderate drug abusers maximally benefit from a referral to a brief intervention as opposed to receiving either a lesser intensive or more intensive treatment option. Finally, testing the IHS-PESQ in other American Indian youth samples will help to judge the generalizability of this screening measure in more diverse native youth populations.

In sum, favorable psychometric findings were obtained in all gender and age subgroups of the American Indian youth groups tested. Accurate screening is essential for the success of the AODAPS given the tool's central role in determining drug intervention needs of Indian youth suspected of drug involvement. The study findings provide preliminary support for this model that attempts to distinguish mild/moderate drug-abusing cases from those at the severe end of the problem severity spectrum.

REFERENCES

Beauvais, F. (1992). Comparison of drug use rates for reservation Indian, non-reservation Indian and Anglo youth. *American Indian and Alaska Native Mental Health Research, 5,* 13-31.

Center for Substance Abuse Treatment. (1999). *Treatment of Adolescents with Substance Use Disorders.* Treatment Improvement Protocol (TIP) Series, Number 32. DHHS Pub. No. (SMA) 99-3283. Washington, D.C.: U.S. Government Printing Office.

Crowne, D.P., & Marlowe, D. (1960). A new scale of social desirability independent of psychopathology. *Journal of Consulting Psychology, 24,* 349-354.

Fry, E. (1977). Fry's readability graph: Clarifications, validity, and extension to level 17. *Journal of Reading, 21,* 242-253.

Henly, G.A. & Winters, K.C. (1988). Development of problem severity scales for the assessment of adolescent alcohol and drug abuse. *The International Journal of the Addictions, 23,* 65-85.

Institute of Medicine. (1990). *Broadening the base of treatment for alcohol problems.* Washington, DC: National Academy Press.

Johnston, L.D., Bachman, J.G, & O'Malley, P.M. (1985). *Monitoring the Future: Questionnaire Responses from the Nation's High School Seniors, 1984.* Ann Arbor, MI: Survey Research Center, Institute for Social Research.

Kaminer, Y. (1994). *Adolescent substance abuse.* New York: Plenum Publishing Corporation.

Mail, P.D. & Johnson, S. (1993). Boozing, sniffing, and toking: An overview of the past, present, and future of substance use by American Indians. *American Indian and Alaska Native Mental Health Research, 5,* 1-33.

Moran, J.R., & Reaman, J.A. (2002). Critical issues for substance abuse prevention targeting American Indian youth. *The Journal of Primary Prevention, 22,* 201-233.

Nunnally, J.C. (1967). *Psychometric theory.* New York: McGraw-Hill.

Rahdert, E.R. (Ed.) (1991). *The Adolescent Assessment/Referral System Manual.* Rockville, MD: U.S. Department of Health and Human Services.

Walker, R.D., Lambert, M.D., Walker, P.S., Klvlahan, D.R., Donovan, D.M. & Howard, M.O. (1996). Alcohol abuse in urban Indian adolescents and women: A longitudinal study for assessment and risk evaluation. *American Indian and Alaska Native Mental health Research, 7,* 1-47.

Weinberg, N. Z., Rahdert, E., Colliver, J. D., & Glantz, M. D. (1998). Adolescent substance abuse: A review of the past 10 years. *Journal of the American Academy of Child & Adolescent Psychiatry, 37,* 252-261.

Williams, R., & Chang, S. (2000). A comprehensive and comparative review of adolescent substance abuse treatment outcome. *Clinical Psychology: Science and Practice, 7,* 138-166.

Winters, K. C. (1992). Development of an adolescent alcohol and other drug abuse screening scale: Personal Experience Screening Questionnaire. *Addictive Behaviors, 17,* 479-490.

Winters, K.C. (1991). *Personal Experience Screening Questionnaire test and manual.* Los Angeles: Western Psychological Services.

Winters, K. C. (1999). Treating adolescents with substance use disorders: An overview of practice issues and treatment outcomes. *Substance Abuse, 20,* 203-225.
Winters, K.C. & Botzet, A. (2002). *Report on drug abuse among American Indian students: Year 2002.* Minneapolis: Center for Substance Abuse Research, University of Minnesota
Winters, K.C. & Henly, G.A. (1988). *Personal Experience Inventory and Manual.* Los Angeles: Western Psychological Services.

doi:10.1300/J029v16n01_04

Adolescent Alcohol and Marijuana Use: Concordance Among Objective-, Self-, and Collateral-Reports

Joseph A. Burleson
Yifrah Kaminer

SUMMARY. The association of and difference between urinalysis, self- and parent collateral-report of alcohol and substance use at baseline, 3- and 9-month follow-up was assessed for 88 male and female adolescents from a treatment study. While urinalyses rates were higher than self- and collateral-report, urinalyses and self-report did not differ significantly at follow-up. Associations between urinalyses and self-report were highest (r = .64, .69), followed by youth-/collateral report (.49, .55), and urinalyses/collateral-report (.28, .43). Change in youth subjective substance use was associated with collateral subjective perceptions of use at follow-up. Higher false-negatives render collateral less reliable than self-report but necessary in the assessment process. doi:10.1300/J029v16n01_05 *[Article copies available for a fee from The Haworth Document Delivery Service: 1-800-HAWORTH. E-mail address: <docdelivery@haworthpress.com> Website: <http://www.HaworthPress.com> © 2006 by The Haworth Press, Inc. All rights reserved.]*

Joseph A. Burleson, PhD, is Assistant Professor in the Department of Community Medicine and Health Care, and Yifrah Kaminer, MD, is Professor in the Department of Psychiatry, both at The University of Connecticut Health Center, Farmington, CT 06030-2103.

This research was supported by grant DA00262-01 to Yifrah Kaminer, Principal Investigator, from the National Institute on Drug Abuse.

[Haworth co-indexing entry note]: "Adolescent Alcohol and Marijuana Use: Concordance Among Objective-, Self-, and Collateral-Reports." Burleson, Joseph A., and Yifrah Kaminer. Co-published simultaneously in *Journal of Child & Adolescent Substance Abuse* (The Haworth Press, Inc.) Vol. 16, No. 1, 2006, pp. 53-68; and: *Adolescent Substance Abuse: New Frontiers in Assessment* (ed: Ken C. Winters) The Haworth Press, Inc., 2006, pp. 53-68. Single or multiple copies of this article are available for a fee from The Haworth Document Delivery Service [1-800-HAWORTH, 9:00 a.m. - 5:00 p.m. (EST). E-mail address: docdelivery@haworthpress.com].

KEYWORDS. Adolescent, substance abuse, alcohol abuse, assessment, urinalysis, treatment

The assessment of youth with either suspected substance use or known substance use disorder (SUD) has classically been accomplished by procuring adolescent self-report (Substance Abuse and Mental Health Services Administration, 1999). Relying solely on adolescent self-report, however, is certain to result in data whose reliability is limited. Most adolescents are at least somewhat coerced into screening or assessment of their substance use, particularly when a decision regarding their need for treatment is waiting. In addition, when adolescents are referred for substance use assessment with the anticipation that they will have to enroll in a treatment program if their levels of use are sufficiently high, the majority does not perceive their levels of use as severe enough to warrant an intervention, and, consequently, are reluctant to cooperate fully (Kaminer, 1994). Self-reports may, however, provide reliable and valid information, particularly when no legal contingencies for drug use are pending (Barnea et al., 1987).

There is a long-standing and general consensus that both parent and child integrated input is ideal for a best-estimate clinical diagnosis of the child (Leckman et al., 1982; Rutter, 1989). To the extent that there is good agreement between child and collateral informant diagnostic information, confidence increases in the validity of the assessment (Cantwell et al., 1997). The limited data available on this topic provide a mixed picture revealing a considerable range of parent-adolescent agreement. The association between different sources of diagnostic information, however, has often been found to be low (Edelbrock et al., 1986). Parent-child concordance has been shown to vary, for example, as a function of disorder type (Achenbach et al., 1987). Concordance is generally high in assessing externalizing versus internalizing problems, presumably because the former are more easily observable.

Youth have reported significantly more internalizing symptoms and more alcohol and drug abuse than their parents report being aware of (Achenbach et al., 1987; Andrews et al., 1993). Cantwell and colleagues (1997) examined the degree of agreement between parent and adolescent report of child major psychiatric disorders. The k values for parent-adolescent agreement on the disorders averaged from 0.19 for alcohol abuse/dependence, 0.41 for substance abuse/dependence, to 0.79 for conduct disorder. Agreement was not influenced by gender, current adolescent age, age of onset of the disorder, or severity of the disorder.

Regional studies reveal that between 7-10% of adolescents are in need of treatment (Harrison et al., 1998; Lewinsohn et al., 1996). Only a small segment of this group, in particular, those with high severity of substance use disorders, comorbid psychiatric disorders, and legal problems, end up in treatment due to limited resources, inadequate age-appropriate quality programs, and lack of a broad consensus on preferred treatment strategies (Kaminer, 2001).

Edelbrock et al. (1986) reported an average mother-child agreement of 63% for SUD symptoms, whereas Weissman et al. (1987) reported an average agreement of 17% for SUD symptoms. Winters et al. (1996) found a modest agreement (r = .35) on a scale measuring personal consequences of drug use. In a more recent study, Winters et al. (2000) reported moderate agreement (r = .27) between mother and child on the drug involvement severity scales. Mothers, however, tended to underreport their child's level of drug involvement and resulting problems compared to child's self-report.

A Partnership for a Drug Free America community survey (CESAR, 1996) stressed the low levels of agreement between child and parental reports of SUD. Adolescent-reported rates of SUD were much higher than parent-reported rates. Similarly, O'Donnell et al. (1998) reported that SUD rates vary by informant and were higher when the child, rather than the parent, was the reporter. Parental reports were frequently endorsed by the child's report, whereas the converse was rarely true. Andrews et al. (1993) identified that parent-child concordance was mediated by the extent to which the adolescent perceived the behavior as socially acceptable.

One clear methodological limitation of most studies exploring this issue has been lack of objective confirmation of SUD, namely, via urinalysis. While the sample size in the present study precluded examining other factors (e.g., gender) that might moderate parent-adolescent concordance, the urinalyses findings allow us to compare each rating with objective measures. Hence, the concordance among objective assessment, youth self-report, and parent collateral-report of youth's substance use was assessed for a group of adolescent substance users.

METHODS

Subjects

The study included 88 adolescents consecutively referred to an outpatient treatment program from 1996 to 1998 for psychoactive substance use disorders (American Psychiatric Association, 1987). The cohort included 62 males, 26 females, ages 13 to 18 years (mean 15.4, SD 1.3 years), of which 79 were white, and 76 of whom completed the program (further details can be found in Kaminer, Burleson, & Goldberger, 2002). Exclusion criteria included: requirement for a more intensive treatment than offered in this study; current acute psychosis or any other psychiatric or medical condition that could interfere with treatment (e.g., poor compliance with medications for ADHD, suicidal or aggressive behavior in the last 30 days); reading and comprehension levels below fifth grade; refusal to consent for either randomization to treatment conditions or for session videotaping; no permanent address; or transportation difficulties for treatment program.

Procedures

A trained research assistant described the study to the subjects and caretakers, and a written, IRB approved informed consent was obtained. Treatment was provided at no cost, and participants and caretaker were compensated for the assessments. Participants completed a baseline assessment battery and were then randomized into one of two closed-group conditions: CBT (n = 51) or PET (n = 37). The 8-week therapy curriculum was composed of 75-90 minute weekly sessions. In order to improve familiarity and compliance with the treatment condition, patients received an introductory section during the first session of their respective treatment conditions. A pair of therapists, from a pool of five doctoral level and master level clinicians experienced in working with adolescents and specifically trained in conducting CBT and PET, was assigned to each treatment condition. That is, each pair provided treatment in both CBT and PET cycles, minimizing therapist variability.

Assessment Instruments

Teen Addiction Severity Index (Kaminer, Bukstein, & Tarter, 1991). This semistructured interview was modified from the Addiction Severity Index (McLellan, Luborsky, Woody, & O'Brien, 1980) to fill the need for a reliable, valid, and standardized instrument for evaluating the severity of adolescent substance abuse and associated problem domains. The T-ASI was found to have good psychometric properties (Kaminer, Wagner, Plummer, & Seifer, 1993). The values of the T-ASI range from zero (no problem) to 4 (major problem).

Urinalysis. Random urinalysis procedures for cannabinoid, cocaine, and opiates were employed during treatment. In addition, all subjects were tested upon treatment completion and follow-ups for a total of three times (EZ-Screen Test Kit; Editek Inc.; Burlington, NC). This qualitative screening essay has shown high specificity and sensitivity to the drugs tested (Kranzler, Stone, & McLaughlin, 1995). The percentage of urines testing positive from among those collected during the treatment sessions was calculated. This skewed variable was dichotomized to represent those who tested positive at all versus those who tested negative throughout therapy. The 3- and 9-M urinalysis results were analyzed as dichotomies.

Data Analysis

The three sets of dichotomous variables concerning youths' marijuana use (parents' subjective assessment, youths' subjective assessment, and objective urinalysis) were assessed at each of the two follow-up time points (3- and 9-months), while two sets of continuous variables concerning youths' alcohol use (parents' subjective assessment, and youths' subjective assessment) were assessed. McNemar's test was used to test the difference between paired rates (i.e., 3-M Youth Self-Report versus 3-M Parent Report). Pearson correlation coefficients were calculated to show the association between all variables, regardless of type (and in order to assess concordance among pairs of dichotomous variables; values of Pearson's r were all within .01 of Cohen's κ, a measure of concordance). Other statistics for the association of two dichotomous variables include the marginal rates of subjective and objective assessments; the sensitivity, specificity, and predictive positive value of the subjective perceptions assessed against the objective or subjective measures. All reported significance tests are 1-tailed, with the exception of the analyses of changes in T-ASI, since only positive correlations were hypothesized; all negative correlations, therefore, regardless of strength, were rejected. For the Pearson correlation, F-, and t-tests, error degrees of freedom (df) are reported in parentheses.

RESULTS

Means and standard deviations (or percentages and sample sizes) are reported in Table 1 for all variables.

TABLE 1. Descriptive Statistics for and Correlations Among Youth and Parent Collateral Measures of Youth Substance and Alcohol Use

Measures	Descriptive Statistics M% a	SD(n) b	Urinalysis DT	3-M	9-M	Marijuana 3-M	9-M	Alcohol 3-M	9-M	Substance BL	3-M	9-M	T-ASI BL	Alcohol 3-M	9-M	Parent: Youth Used Substance 3-M	9-M	Alcohol 3-M	9-M	Parent T-ASI Substance 3-M	9-M	Alcohol 3-M
Youth																						
Urinalysis (% +)																						
During Tx	46.1%	(41)	-													-	-	-	-	-	-	-
3-M	43.3%	(26)	.27*	-												-	-	-	-	-	-	-
9-M	58.0%	(29)	.27*	.19	-											-	-	-	-	-	-	-
Used marijuana																						
3-M	36.2%	(25)	.24*	.69**	.42**	-										-	-	-	-	-	-	-
9-M	41.8%	(23)	.14	.42*	.64**	.58**	-									-	-	-	-	-	-	-
Used alcohol																						
3-M	27.5%	(19)	.06	.05	.32*	.21*	.17	-								-	-	-	-	-	-	-
9-M	49.1%	(27)	.27*	.02	.28*	.09	.27*	.42**	-							-	-	-	-	-	-	-
T-ASI-substance																						
Baseline	1.5	-1.0/1.3	.12	.01	.13	.12	.30*	.05	-.05	-						-	-	-	-	-	-	-
3-M	0.4	-0.4/1.2	.16+	.52**	.07	.46**	.25*	.04	-.01	.22*	-					-	-	-	-	-	-	-
9-M	0.3	-0.3/1.0	.14	.32*	.55**	.51**	.64**	.23+	.23+	.24*	.38*	-				-	-	-	-	-	-	-
T-ASI-alcohol																						
Baseline	0.7	-0.7/1.4	-.07	-.07	-.12	-.16	.03	.20+	.08	.22*	.01	.04	-			-	-	-	-	-	-	-
3-M	0.2	-0.2/0.8	.01	-.03	-.06	-.05	-.03	.20*	.16	.06	.32**	.16	.40**	-		-	-	-	-	-	-	-
9-M	0.2	-0.2/0.5	.16	.12	.15	.05	.02	.23*	.66**	-.21	.04	.17	.07	.29*	-	-	-	-	-	-	-	-

Parent collateral

Used marijuana																							
3-M	36.4%	(24)	.01	.28*	.31*	.49**	.50**	.19+	.07	.10	.15	.46**	.10	.15	−.04	−						
9-M	30.8%	(16)	.19+	.19	.43**	.35**	.55**	.18	.15	.09	.17	.60**	.03	.04	.10	.33*	−					
Used alcohol																							
3-M	17.8%	(19)	−.18	−.17	.26+	.01	.15	.46**	.33**	.08	−.04	.25*	.22*	.36*	.20+	.22*	.18	−				
9-M	36.5%	(19)	−.01	.14	.18	.15	.18	.18	.42**	−.02	.28*	.21+	.11	.30*	.45**	.16	.19+	−				
T-ASI-substance																							
3-M	1.0	−0.9/1.7	−.10	.33**	.19	.28*	.36**	.11	.15	.16	.45**	.32*	.39**	.29**	.11	.47**	.29*	.10	.10	−		
9-M	0.7	−0.7/1.7	.02	.40**	.31*	.28*	.51**	.00	.23+	−.07	.32*	.57**	.15	.30*	.17	.23+	.56**	.21+	.37**	.36**	−	
T-ASI-alcohol																							
3-M	0.7	−0.7/1.4	−.18+	.09	.10	−.00	.28*	.22*	.41**	.13	.19+	.20+	.60**	.51**	.30*	.14	.25*	.42**	.29*	.63**	.46**	−
9-M	0.5	−0.5/1.3	−.08	.31*	.15	.08	.26*	−.07	.18	−.02	.40**	.28*	.24*	.40**	.35**	.17	.31*	.29*	.57**	.38**	.56**	.46**

[a] Note that listed rates differ slightly depending on the concordance analysis sample size
[b] +SD/−SD Note that standard deviations are not symmetrical due to use of linear transformation of data
+ p < .10
* p < .05
** p < .01

Urinalysis and Youth Self-Report

There was no significant difference between the 3-M urinalysis rate (42.4%) and the 3-M Youth Self-Report rate (33.9%), p = .18 (the base rates reported in Table 1 reflect the maximum number of cases, and are slightly different). There was, however, a significant association between 3-M Youth Self-Report and 3-M urinalysis, r(57) = .69, p < .001. Using the urinalysis as the standard, OR = 41.14, χ^2 = 28.11, Positive Predictive Value (PPV) = .90, Negative Predictive Value (NPV) = .82, Sensitivity (Se) = .72, Specificity (Sp) = .94 (as shown in Table 2). There was also no significant difference between the 9-M urinalysis rate (57.4%) and the 9-M Youth Self-Report rate (46.8%), p = .18. There was, however, also a significant association between 9-M Youth Self-Report and 9-M urinalysis, r(45) = .64, p < .001, OR = 25.71, χ^2 = 18.95, PPV = .74, NPV = .90, Se = .91, Sp = .72.

Urinalysis and Youth T-ASI

The BL T-ASI Substance subscale was not significantly associated with any of the three urinalyses (DT, 3-M, 9-M), nor was the DT urinalysis significantly associated with any of the Substance subscales at any of the three assessment times. However, the 3-M urinalysis was significantly associated with both the 3-M, r(57) = .52, p < .001, and the 9-M T-ASI Substance subscales, r(57) = .32, p = .016. The 9-M T-ASI Substance subscale was significantly associated with the 9-M urinalysis, r(45) = .55, p < .001. As might be expected, both time-concordant associations were significantly higher than the time discordant correlations.

Urinalyses and Parent Collateral Report

Neither the 3- nor 9-M Parent Substance Collateral Report was significantly associated with the DT urinalyses. There was no significant difference between the 3-M urinalysis rate (41.8%) and the 3-M Parent Collateral-Report rate (36.4%), p = .65. However, the 3-M Parent Substance Collateral Report was significantly associated with the 3-M urinalyses, r(53) = .28, p = .039. Using the urinalysis as the standard, OR = 3.27, χ^2 = 4.27, PPV = .60, NPV = .69, Se = .52, Sp = .75. There was, however, a significant difference between the 9-M urinalysis rate (56.8%) and the 9-M Parent Collateral-Report rate (34.1%), p = .013. The 9-M Parent Substance Collateral Report was also significantly as-

TABLE 2. Odds, Predicted Values, Sensitivity, and Specificity for Time-Concordant Dichotomous Measures

Test/Standard variable	n	χ^2	p	Odds	PPV	NPV	Sens	Spec
Youth Self-Report Substance/Urinalysis								
3-M	59	28.11	<.001	41.14	.90	.82	.72	.94
9-M	47	18.95	<.001	25.71	.74	.90	.91	.72
Parent Collateral-Report Substance/Urinalysis								
3-M	55	4.27	.039	3.27	.60	.69	.52	.75
9-M	44	8.26	.004	9.21	.87	.59	.52	.90
Parent Collateral-Report/Youth Self-Report								
Alcohol								
3-M	63	13.19	<.001	8.71	.58	.86	.65	.83
9-M	47	8.08	.004	6.50	.77	.67	.57	.83
Substance								
3-M	63	15.21	<.001	9.14	.67	.82	.70	.80
9-M	47	14.06	<.001	16.61	.87	.72	.59	.92

sociated with the 9-M urinalyses, $r(42) = .43$, $p = .004$, as would be expected. Using the urinalysis as the standard, $OR = 9.21$, $\chi^2 = 8.26$, PPV $= .87$, NPV $= .59$, Se $= .52$, Sp $= .90$. Only one time-discordant association was significant, however, the 3-M Parent Substance/Youth 9-M urinalysis, $r(45) = .31$, $p = .036$.

Urinalyses and Parent Collateral T-ASI

Neither the 3- nor 9-M Parent Substance subscale was significantly associated with the DT urinalyses. However, both time-concordant associations were significantly associated with urinalyses, 3-M $r(54) = .33$, $p = .006$; 9-M $r(42) = .31$, $p = .02$, as would be expected. Only one time-discordant association was significant, however, the 9-M Parent Substance subscale/Youth 3-M urinalysis, $r(44) = .40$, $p = .003$.

Youth Self-Report and Parent Collateral-Report

Alcohol. There was no significant difference between the 3-M Youth Self-Report rate (27.0%) and the 3-M Parent Collateral-Report rate (30.2%), $p = .79$. There was, however, a significant association between 3-M Youth Alcohol Self-Report and Parent Collateral-Report of Alcohol Use, $r(61) = .46$, $p < .001$. Using the Youth Self-Report as the standard, $OR = 8.71$, $\chi^2 = 13.19$, PPV $= .58$, NPV $= .86$, Se $= .65$, Sp $= .83$. There was also no significant difference between the 9-M Youth Self-Report rate (48.9%) and the 9-M Parent Collateral-Report rate (36.2%), $p = .18$. There was, however, a significant association between 9-M Youth Self-Report and Parent Collateral-Report, $r(45) = .42$, $p = .004$. Using the Youth Self-Report as the standard, $OR = 6.50$, $\chi^2 = 8.08$, PPV $= .77$, NPV $= .67$, Se $= .57$, Sp $= .83$.

Substance. There was no significant difference between the 3-M Youth Self-Report rate (36.5%) and the 3-M Parent Collateral-Report rate (38.1%), $p = 1.00$. There was, however, a significant association between 3-M Youth Substance Self-Report and Parent Collateral-Report of Substance Use, $r(61) = .49$, $p < .001$. Using the Youth Self-Report as the standard, $OR = 9.14$, $\chi^2 = 15.21$, PPV $= .67$, NPV $= .82$, Se $= .70$, Sp $= .80$. There was a trend toward a significant difference between the 9-M Youth Self-Report rate (46.8%) and the 9-M Parent Collateral-Report rate (31.9%), $p = .065$, with the youth reporting a higher rate. There was also a significant association between 9-M Youth Self-Report and Parent Collateral-Report, $r(45) = .55$, $p < .001$. Using the Youth Self-Report as the standard, OR = 16.61, χ^2 = 14.06, PPV = .87, NPV = .72, Se = .59, Sp = .92.

Youth T-ASI and Parent Collateral T-ASI

Generally, associations between parent and youth were higher for same subscales (e.g., both Alcohol or both Substance), and associations were as high or slightly higher for concordant time points (e.g., both 3-M). However, the Parent-Youth Alcohol associations were somewhat higher at BL and at 3-M, with Substance associations somewhat higher at 9-M.

Alcohol. Parent-Youth Alcohol associations were significant for all time points, 3-M r(62) = .51, p < .001; and 9-M r(47) = .35, p = .008. The Youth BL was highly associated with Parent 3-M, 3-M r(64) = .60, p < .001, possibly because parents had become aware of their child's reported BL levels by then. By 9-M, however, this effect was attenuated, 9-M r(50) = .24, p = .043.

Substance. Parent-Youth Alcohol associations were significant for all time points, especially Youth BL with Parent 3-M r(62) = .45, p < .001; and Youth BL with Parent 9-M r(47) = .57, p < .001. Contrary to the Alcohol result, the Youth BL was not significantly associated with Parent 3- and 9-M.

T-TASI Change from Baseline

Alcohol 3-M. The youth 3-M T-ASI Alcohol subscale was significantly positively associated with Youth Baseline T-ASI Alcohol subscale at the first entry step in the sequential regression, F(1,62) = 12.46, p = .001, Δr^2 = .17. The final equation does not show Baseline to be significant, however, β = .15, t(61) = 1.04, p = .30. The change in the youth Alcohol subscale from BL to 3-M was significantly associated with the Parent 3-M Alcohol subscale at entry, F(1,61) = 8.58, p = .005, Δr^2 = .10, and remains significant in the final equation, standardized β = .41, t(61) = 2.93, p = .005, such that the better the Parental score (low value), the better the Youth score. Youths' positive change at 3-months is associated with parents' positive perceptions at 3-months.

Alcohol 9-M. The youth 9-M T-ASI Alcohol subscale, however, was not significantly associated with Youth Baseline T-ASI Alcohol subscale at the first entry step, F(1,43) = 0.00, p = .99, Δr^2 = .00. Nonetheless, the change in the youth Alcohol subscale from BL to 9-M showed a trend toward significance with Parent 3-M Alcohol subscale at entry, $F(1,42) = 3.91$, $p = .055$, $\Delta r^2 = .09$, as it did with Parent 9-M Alcohol subscale at entry, $F(1,41) = 3.02$, $p = .09$, $\Delta r^2 = .06$. The final equation shows a trend toward significance only for this last Parent 9-M Alcohol subscale, standardized $\beta = .28$, $t(41) = 1.74$, $p = .09$, such that the better the Parental score, the better the Youth score. Youths' positive change at 9-months is associated with parents' positive perceptions at 9-months. Neither Youth Baseline, standardized $\beta = -.19$, $t(41) = -1.03$, $p = 31$, nor for Parent 3-M Alcohol subscale, standardized $\beta = .22$, $t(41) = 1.07$, $p = .29$, were significant in the final equation.

Substance 3-M. The youth 3-M T-ASI Substance subscale showed a trend toward significance for a positive association with Youth Baseline T-ASI Substance subscale at the first entry step, $F(1,62) = 3.59$, $p = .063$, $\Delta r^2 = .06$. The change in the Substance subscale from BL to 3-M was significantly associated with Parent 3-M Substance at entry, $F(1,61) = 14.11$, $p < .001$, $\Delta r^2 = .18$. The final equation shows significance only for this latter Parent 3-M Substance subscale, standardized $\beta = .43$, $t(61) = 3.76$, $p < .001$, such that the better the Parental score, the better the Youth score. Youths' positive change at 3-months is associated with parents' positive perceptions at 3-months. Youth Baseline was not significant in the final equation, standardized $\beta = .17$, $t(61) = 1.53$, $p = .13$.

Substance 9-M. The youth 9-M T-ASI Substance subscale was not significantly associated with Youth Baseline T-ASI Substance subscale at the first entry step, $F(1,43) = 0.97$, $p = .33$, $\Delta r^2 = .02$. Nonetheless, this change from BL to 9-M was significantly associated with Parent 3-M Substance, $F(1,42) = 5.74$, $p = .021$, $\Delta r^2 = .12$, and with Parent 9-M Substance, $F(1,41) = 18.20$, $p < .001$, $\Delta r^2 = .26$. The final equation shows significance only for this latter Parent 9-M Substance subscale, standardized $\beta = .56$, $t(41) = 4.27$, $p < .001$, such that the better the Parental score, the better the Youth score. Youths' positive change at 9-months is associated with parents' positive perceptions at 9-months. Neither Youth Baseline, standardized $\beta = .20$, $t(41) = 1.64$, $p = .11$, nor Parent 3-M Substance subscale, standardized $\beta = .12$, $t(41) = 0.93$, $p = .36$, were significant in the final equation.

DISCUSSION

The purpose of this study was to examine the parent-child subjective agreement, as well as agreement with objective results (i.e., drug urinalysis) for adolescents with SUD in an outpatient program. As might be expected, the agreement between urinalysis and youth self-report, while moderate, was higher than any agreement with parental assessments. While both of the youth subjective self-report measures examined showed high agreement with urinalysis, the direct, single-item statement concerning use showed higher agreement than did the T-ASI Substance Use subscale. This might be expected since the three items that comprise the T-ASI Substance Use subscale do not explicitly address the youth's current use as such. Accordingly, the youth subjective self-report was more highly associated with urinalysis than was parent subjective self-report. Independent of the level of agreement, there was also no significant difference between urinalyses and youth self-report rates. While there was no significant difference between urinalysis and parent collateral-report at 3-months, there was a significant difference at 9-months. Finally, as might be expected, any particular association between urinalyses and substance use was almost always significantly higher than the analogous association between urinalyses and alcohol use.

With the exception of a trend for 9-month substance use, there were no significant differences between the subjective youth versus parent reported use of either alcohol or other substances. Separate from the urinalyses, the agreement between parent and youth subjective measures was of similar strength regardless of whether substance use or alcohol use was assessed. Since less agreement might be expected concerning illegal substance use due to associated social admonitions and legal risks, the similarity of substance use and alcohol use agreement is noteworthy.

Agreement between parent and youth subjective reports was similar for 3-M versus 9-M. For assessments of substance use, however, the 9-M agreements were higher. For alcohol agreement, on the other hand, there was not a clear pattern, with either 3- or 9-M agreements being higher, depending on the two measures being assessed. It might be assumed that as both parent and youth are exposed to and become familiar with being asked to make these assessments, that they might, over time, increase their rate of concordance. This convergence over time may have happened concerning substance use, but was not evident with assessments of alcohol use. Again, as might be expected, any particular association between substance use and alcohol use was almost always significantly lower than either of the analogous associations within substance and within alcohol use.

In assessing whether parental perceptions of their child's functional status might predict the *change* in the youth's perceptions of their functional status, it was seen that for both alcohol and other substance measures, and at both 3- and 9-months, parents' perceptions significantly predicted the change in youth's status, with the higher the parent's subsequent view of the youth, the more progress the youth perceived him/ herself to have made. This analysis of change, however, would need to be based on a larger sample size, with other, concomitant measures taken in addition. It is logical, however, to imagine that parents might be sensitive to the change in their child's perceived status, despite their underestimation of their child's substance use.

There was no clear pattern of differences between use of the dichotomous Use/Non-Use variable versus the continuous T-ASI subjective scale measures in assessing concordance between parent and youth substance use when, nor were there any analogous differences in concordance when assessing alcohol use.

Relative to the two studies cited which compared concordance for SUD *symptoms*, our concordance rates for substance use *per se*, while high, are generally lower than the r = .63 found by Edelbrock et al. (1986), and substantially higher than the κ = .17 found by Weissman et al. (1987). Relative to Cantwell et al.'s (1997) concordance for substance *dependence*, our rates are comparable.

The present results showing that youth report more substance use than their parents perceive are consistent with literature suggesting that parents may often be unaware of the general recent history, as well as the specificity, frequency, and magnitude of their children's substance use. Between 95-100% of adolescent alcohol and other substance abuse are identified by the adolescent's report. Presumably for these disorders, parent report identifies very few additional cases (Cantwell et al., 1997). If forced to choose between the adolescent and the parent, relying on the adolescent report would appear, therefore, to result in the detection of more diagnosed cases (Cantwell et al., 1997). Nonetheless, Winters et al. (2000) state that despite the severe deficits in parental knowledge regarding their children's substance use, parent collateral report is still a desirable source of information that may allow functional assessment of other life domains, legal consequences, and potential treatment outcomes.

REFERENCES

Achenbach, T. M., McConaughy, S. H., & Howell, C. T. (1987). Child/adolescent behavioral and emotional problems: Implications of cross-informant correlations for situational specificity. *Psychological Bulletin, 101*, 213-232.

American Psychiatric Association (1987). *Diagnostic and statistical manual of mental disorders* (Third Edition-Revised). Washington, DC: American Psychiatric Association.

Andrews, V. C., Garrison, C. Z., Jackson, K. L., Addy, C. L., & McKeown, R. E. (1993). Mother-adolescent agreement on the symptoms and diagnoses of adolescent depression and conduct disorders. *Journal of the American Academy of Child and Adolescent Psychiatry, 32*, 731-738.

Barnea, A., Rahav, G., & Teichman, M. (1987). The reliability and consistency of self-reports of substance use in a longitudinal study. *British Journal of Addictions, 82*, 891-898.

Cantwell, D. P., Lewinsohn, P. M., Rohde, P., & Seeley, J. R. (1997). Correspondence between adolescent report and parent report of psychiatric diagnostic data. *Journal of the American Academy of Child and Adolescent Psychiatry, 36*, 610-619.

Center for Substance Abuse Treatment. (1999). *Screening and assessing adolescents for substance use disorders.* Treatment Improvement Protocol (TIP) Series, Number 31. DHHS Publication No. (SMA) 99-3344. Washington, DC: U. S. Government Printing Office.

CESAR (1996). Poll shows that patients seriously underestimate availability and use of drugs among their children. *Partnership for a Drug Free America, 5*(16). College Park, MD: University of Maryland.

Edelbrock, C., & Achenbach, T. M. (1986). A typology of child behavior profile patterns: Distribution and correlates for disturbed children age 6 to 16. *Journal of Abnormal Child Psychology, 8*, 441-470.

Harrison, P. A., Fulkerson, J. A., & Beebe, T. J. (1998). DSM-IV substance use disorder criteria for adolescents: A critical examination based on a statewide school survey. *American Journal of Psychiatry, 155*, 486-492.

Kaminer, Y. (1994). *Adolescent substance abuse: A comprehensive guide to theory and practice.* New York: Plenum Press.

Kaminer, Y. (2001). Adolescent substance abuse treatment: Where do we go from here? *Psychiatric Services, 52*, 147-149.

Kaminer, Y., Bukstein, O. G., & Tarter, R. E. (1991). The Teen Addiction Severity Index: Rationale and reliability. *International Journal of the Addictions, 26*, 219-226.

Kaminer, Y., Burleson, J. A., & Goldberger, R. (2002). Psychotherapies for adolescent substance abusers: Short- and long-term outcomes. *Journal of Nervous and Mental Disease, 190*: 737-745.

Kaminer, Y., Wagner, E., Plummer, B., & Seifer, R. (1993). Validation of the Teen Addiction Severity Index: Preliminary findings. *American Journal of Addiction, 2*, 221-224.

Kranzler, H. R., Stone, J., & McLaughlin, L. (1995). Evaluation of a point-of-care testing product for drugs of abuse: Testing site is a key variable. *Drug and Alcohol Dependence, 40*, 55-62.

Leckman, J., Sholomskas, D., & Thompson, W. (1982). Best estimate of lifetime psychiatric diagnosis: A methodological study. *Archives of General Psychiatry, 39,*
879-883.

Lewinsohn, P. M., Rohde, P., & Seeley, J. (1996). Alcohol consumption in high school
adolescents: Frequency of use and dimensional structure of associated problems.
Addiction, 91, 375-390.

McLellan, A. T., Luborsky, L., Woody, G. E., & O'Brien, C. P. (1980). An improved
diagnostic evaluation instrument for substance abuse patients. *Journal of Nervous
and Mental Disease, 173,* 412-423.

O'Donnell, D., Biederman, J., Jones, J., Wilens, T. E., Milberger, S., Mick, E., &
Varaone, S. V. (1998). Informativeness of child and parent reports on substance use
disorders in a sample of ADHD probands, control probands, and their siblings.
Journal of the American Academy of Child and Adolescent Psychiatry, 37, 752-758.

Rutter, M. (1989). Isle of Wight revisited: Twenty-five years of child psychiatric epidemiology. *Journal of the American Academy of Child and Adolescent Psychiatry,
28,* 633-653.

Weissman, M. M., Wickramaratne, P., Warner, V., John, K., Prusoff, B. A., Meri-
kangas, K. R., & Gammon, D. (1987). Assessing psychiatric disorders in children:
Discrepancies between mother's and children's reports. *Archives of General Psychiatry, 44,* 747, 753.

Winters, K. C., Anderson, N., Bengston, P., Stinchfield, R. D., & Latimer, W. W.
(2000). Development of a parent questionnaire for use in assessing adolescent drug
abuse. *Journal of Psychoactive Drugs, 32,* 3-13.

Winters, K. C., Stinchfield, R., & Henly, G. A. (1996). Convergent and predictive validity of scales measuring adolescent substance abuse. *Journal of Child & Adolescent Substance Abuse, 5,* 37-55.

doi:10.1300/J029v16n01_05

Adolescent Substance Abuse in Mexico, Puerto Rico and the United States: Effect of Anonymous versus Confidential Survey Formats

William W. Latimer
Megan S. O'Brien
Marco A. Vasquez
Maria Elena Medina-Mora
Carlos F. Rios-Bedoya
Leah J. Floyd

William W. Latimer, PhD, MPH, is Associate Professor and Drs. Megan S. O'Brien and Leah J. Floyd are Postdoctoral Fellows in the Department of Mental Health, Johns Hopkins University, Bloomberg School of Public Health, 624 North Broadway, Baltimore, MD 21205. Marco A. Vasquez is affiliated with the University of Minnesota. Dr. Maria Elena Medina-Mora is Head of the Epidemiological and Social Sciences Department at the Instituto Mexicano de Psiquiatria (IMP), Mexico. Dr. Carlos F. Rios-Bedoya is affiliated with the Ponce School of Medicine, Ponce, Puerto Rico.

Address correspondence to William Latimer, PhD, MPH (E-mail: wlatimer@jhsph.edu.).

The authors would like to acknowledge the epidemiological and statistical support to this paper of the Epidemiology and Biostatistics CORE Program of the Ponce School of Medicine. This CORE Program is federally funded by NIH/NCRR/RCMI Grant Number: 2G12RR03050-18. They would also like to thank O'Malley and colleagues for permission to use Monitoring the Future data. This research was also partially supported by NIDA grant DA00254 to William W. Latimer, PhD, MPH and by the Arthur D. Meyer Award from the University of Minnesota, Division of Epidemiology, School of Public Health.

[Haworth co-indexing entry note]: "Adolescent Substance Abuse in Mexico, Puerto Rico and the United States: Effect of Anonymous versus Confidential Survey Formats." Latimer, William W. et al. Co-published simultaneously in *Journal of Child & Adolescent Substance Abuse* (The Haworth Press, Inc.) Vol. 16, No. 1, 2006, pp. 69-89; and: *Adolescent Substance Abuse: New Frontiers in Assessment* (ed: Ken C. Winters) The Haworth Press, Inc., 2006, pp. 69-89. Single or multiple copies of this article are available for a fee from The Haworth Document Delivery Service [1-800-HAWORTH, 9:00 a.m. - 5:00 p.m. (EST). E-mail address: docdelivery@haworthpress.com].

SUMMARY. Anonymous surveys have been widely used worldwide to describe adolescent substance use yet cannot elucidate causal drug abuse predictors. Studies in the U.S. have generally found that anonymous and confidential surveys yield comparable levels of self-reported substance use, yet the effect of survey format on youth self-report has not been evaluated in other countries. The present study compared data from the confidential International Longitudinal Survey of Adolescent Health with anonymously collected survey data on alcohol and marijuana use among school-based youth in Mexico, Puerto Rico, and the U.S. The findings suggest that confidential surveys yield valid self-reports of adolescent substance use. doi:10.1300/J029v16n01_06 *[Article copies available for a fee from The Haworth Document Delivery Service: 1-800-HAWORTH. E-mail address: <docdelivery@haworthpress.com> Website: <http://www.HaworthPress.com>* © *2006 by The Haworth Press, Inc. All rights reserved.]*

KEYWORDS. Adolescent, anonymous, confidential, cross-cultural, survey, substance abuse

School-based surveys are the most common means whereby epidemiological information on adolescent substance use has been obtained during the past 25 years. In the United States, there are several examples of such national and statewide surveys. Monitoring the Future (MTF) (Johnston, O'Malley, & Bachman, 2002) and the Youth Risk Behavior Surveillance Survey (YRBSS) (Centers for Disease Control and Prevention [CDC], 2002) are two well-known national school-based surveys assessing adolescent substance use. In addition, the majority of states and many school districts conduct their own surveys (Hallfors & Iritani, 2002). Some states, including Iowa and Texas (Iowa Department of Public Health, 2000; Wallisch & Liu, 1998), administer their own surveys while other states choose to administer a modification of a national survey. For example, Rhode Island's Adolescent Substance Abuse Survey (Rhode Island Department of Health, 2000) borrowed many items from the YRBSS to enhance comparability to national data. Similarly, the Maryland Adolescent Survey (Griffith, Loeb, & Dutil, 2001), and the Alcohol, Tobacco, and Other Drug Use by Indiana Children and Adolescents Survey (Indiana Prevention Resource Center, 2002) were modeled after the Monitoring the Future survey study (Johnston, O'Malley, & Bachman, 2002). In addition, commercial surveys, such as the PRIDE Drug Survey, have been used by several states, including Texas (Wallisch & Liu, 1998) and Ohio (Ohio Department of Alcohol and Drug Addiction Services & Ohio Department of Education) and are available for national, state, and local administration.

These national surveys have been instrumental to substance use prevention efforts by providing information on substance use levels among school-based youth. Research comparing self-report of youth substance use to objective methods such as blood tests, has shown that self-report of substance use in adolescents can provide valid information (McNeil et al., 1987; Winters & Henley, 1989). With the exception of the MTF survey administration to 12th grade students, each of the above surveys was anonymous. However, cross-sectional data derived via anonymous survey methods are characterized by important limitations that greatly hamper the ability to identify causal predictors of adolescent drug abuse. Most importantly among these limitations is the inability of cross-sectional data to identify across-time predictors of the onset and severity of adolescent drug abuse. To do so would require both a confidential survey and longitudinal assessment survey procedures. However, the use of confidential rather than anonymous survey procedures raises important methodological and ethical questions. One key methodological question concerns whether youth self-report of sensitive information, such as substance use, is comparable whether information is obtained via anonymous or confidential survey methods. One key ethical question concerns a weighing of adverse events that could result from breaches of confidentiality when students provide identifying information on surveys versus the value of evaluating across-time drug abuse predictors via longitudinal data from a confidential survey.

The methodological issue of the effects of anonymous versus confidential survey formats on youth self-report has been addressed in several studies in the U.S. (Bjarnason & Adalbjarnardottir, 2000; O'Malley, Johnston, Bachman, & Schulenberg, 2000). Generally, the findings suggest that confidential and anonymous methods produce comparable rates of self-reported behaviors by youth, even for sensitive and illegal behaviors. One study comparing anonymous and confidential administrations of the Monitoring the Future survey to 8th and 10th grade students found only negligible differences in the reported use of a variety of substances (O'Malley et al., 2000).

Many countries other than the U.S. have also used anonymous school-based surveys to gauge youth substance use levels. For example, the Alcohol and Other Drug Use Among Students (ESPAD) survey is an anonymous, school-based student survey that has been administered in approximately 30 European countries (Hibell et al., 2000). Two other anonymous school-based surveys conducted outside the U.S. include the National Survey of Drug Use administered in Mexico (Medina-Mora et al., 1992), and the Drug Use Among Adolescent Students survey administered in Puerto Rico (Moscoso, Robles, Colon, & Garcia, 1998).

However, international studies evaluating the effects of survey format on adolescent self-report are lacking (Bjarnason & Adalbjarnardottir, 2000). The present study was an initial attempt to address this gap by comparing substance use frequencies reported by youth in the International Longitudinal Study of Adolescent Health that used a confidential survey format against data obtained by the most recent national studies conducted in Mexico, Puerto Rico, and the U.S. that used anonymous survey formats (Latimer et al., 1999).

METHOD

Study I

Design

The International Longitudinal Survey of Adolescent Health is a multi-wave confidential survey study examining a range of health behaviors, including drug use, sexual behavior, psychiatric problems, and school achievement among school-based youth in Mexico, Puerto Rico, and the United States (Latimer et al. 1999; O'Brien & Latimer, 2002). The present study findings are based on data from the survey administered to one middle school (grades 7-9) and one high school (grades 10-12) in each participating country (i.e., Mexico, Puerto Rico, and the United States) in the spring of 2000. The study survey and procedure were reviewed and approved by each school's Superintendent, an ad hoc review board convened at each participating school comprised of the principal, teachers, and parents, and the University of Minnesota Institutional Review Board.

Participants

All students attending middle school and high school in one community in Mexico, Puerto Rico, and the U.S. were invited to participate in the study. School selection followed similar procedures in each country (e.g., see Latimer et al., 2004).

In Mexico, a total of 1,238 adolescents completed the survey with less than 1% of youth ($n = 9$) excluded from the present study analyses by virtue of either endorsing any use of a fictitious drug item or inconsistent responses throughout the survey. The final sample was comprised of 1,229 youth representing 93% of students enrolled at the participating schools. These 1,229 participants were between 12 and 19 years of age ($M = 15.14$; $SD = 1.71$), with a majority self-identifying as Hispanic (88%) and a slightly higher proportion of females (54%).

In Puerto Rico, a total of 989 adolescents completed the survey with less than 2% of youth ($n = 17$) excluded from the present study analyses by virtue of either endorsing any use of a fictitious drug item or inconsistent responses throughout the survey. The final sample was comprised of 972 youth representing 88% of students enrolled at the participating schools. Similar to the participants in Mexico, these 972 participants were between 11 and 19 years of age ($M = 14.89$; $SD = 1.67$), with a majority self-identifying as Hispanic (96%) and a slightly higher proportion of females (57%).

In the U.S., a total of 1,432 adolescents completed the survey with less than 2% of youth ($n = 26$) excluded from the present study analyses by virtue of either endorsing any use of a fictitious drug item or inconsistent responses throughout the survey. The final sample was comprised of 1,406 youth representing 89% of students enrolled at the participating schools. These 1,406 participants were between 12 and 19 years of age ($M = 14.91$; $SD = 1.67$), with a majority self-identifying as White (91%) and a nearly equal proportion of females (51%) and males. Sample characteristics for each school participating in the International Longitudinal Survey of Adolescent Health are illustrated in Table 1.

Survey Instrument

The Spanish- and English-language versions of the survey were developed over a two-year period (Latimer et al., 1999). Initially, English-language versions of standardized adolescent assessment tools were selected for possible inclusion in the Spanish-language survey. Items on adolescent health and sexuality were derived primarily from the Minnesota Adolescent Health Survey (Latimer, Resnick, & Blum, 1996). Items on adolescent substance use frequency were derived primarily from the Personal Experience Inventory (Winters & Henly, 1989). Items on DSM-IV-defined psychiatric disorders were derived

TABLE 1. Confidential Survey Sample Characteristics*

	Mexico N (%)	Puerto Rico N (%)	United States N (%)
Gender			
Female	659 (53.6)	556 (57.2)	713 (50.7)
Male	570 (46.4)	416 (42.8)	693 (49.3)
Age			
11	000 (00.0)	011 (01.1)	000 (00.0)
12	072 (05.9)	086 (08.8)	067 (04.8)
13	195 (15.9)	126 (13.0)	265 (18.8)
14	184 (15.0)	156 (16.0)	307 (21.8)
15	232 (18.9)	207 (21.3)	268 (19.1)
16	246 (20.0)	202 (20.8)	210 (14.9)
17	195 (15.9)	154 (15.8)	171 (12.2)
18	100 (08.1)	027 (02.8)	115 (08.2)
19	005 (00.4)	003 (00.3)	003 (00.2)
Ethnicity			
Hispanic	1078 (87.7)	932 (95.9)	0021 (01.5)
White	0027 (02.2)	007 (00.7)	1277 (90.8)
Indigenous	0054 (04.4)	009 (00.9)	0002 (00.1)
African American	0006 (00.5)	001 (00.1)	0009 (00.6)
Asian	0000 (00.0)	000 (00.0)	0035 (02.5)
Other	0064 (05.2)	023 (02.4)	0062 (04.4)
Grade			
7	231 (18.8)	167 (17.2)	270 (19.2)
8	187 (15.2)	128 (13.2)	305 (21.7)
9	177 (14.4)	147 (15.1)	267 (19.0)
10	253 (20.6)	181 (18.6)	228 (16.2)
11	193 (15.7)	178 (18.3)	189 (13.4)
12	188 (15.3)	171 (17.6)	147 (10.5)

*Table 1 summarizes characteristics of samples that enrolled in the International Longitudinal Study of Adolescent Health directed by the first author. Detailed characteristics of comparison samples may be found in Johnston, O'Malley, & Bachman, 2002; Medina-Mora, Villatoro, & Rojas, 1996; and Parrilla, Moscoso, Velez, Robles, & Colon, 1997.

mainly from the Adolescent Diagnostic Interview (Winters & Henly, 1993).

Separate forward and backward instrument translation teams based in the United States, Mexico, and Puerto Rico included at least two bilingual allied health professionals in psychology, medicine, public health, or education. Initially, the forward translation teams (one team each in the U.S., Mexico, and Puerto Rico) translated the study instruments from English into Spanish. Next, the backward translation teams translated the Spanish-language versions of tools prepared by the forward teams from Spanish back into English. Following backward translations, the bi-lingual project coordinator developed a draft Spanish-language version of the survey based on the versions provided by each translation team.

The draft version of the Spanish-language survey was subsequently administered to 35 students enrolled in northern Mexico, 17 students enrolled in Puerto Rico, and to seven bilingual Mexican-American adolescents in the United States. Overall, the draft survey appeared to have good face validity; however, minor modifications were made to some survey items following feedback from students completing the draft version.

Substance Use Frequency

Survey items used to ascertain alcohol and marijuana use frequencies were derived from the Personal Experience Inventory (Winters & Henly, 1989). The Personal Experience Inventory has been used extensively in both school and clinic settings with evidence of sound psychometric properties (Winters & Henly, 1989; Winters, Latimer, & Stinchfield, 1999). Survey items on substance use frequency had seven response choices, ranging from never to 40-or-more times, to report substance use during the respondent's lifetime and during 3-month and 12-month periods preceding the survey administration.

Procedure

Following a procedure adapted from the confidential survey methodology used in the Monitoring the Future study (Johnston, O'Malley, Bachman, & Schulenberg, 2000), parents of all students enrolled in the two participating schools in each country were sent a letter describing the study on two separate occasions. These letters were sent three months and two weeks prior to the survey administration date. Less than one percent of parents and less than one percent of students elected not to participate in the survey. One week prior to the survey administration, all teachers in each school received a 3-hour didactic session on how to administer the survey that included printed instructions with verbatim statements for teachers to read to students. The project director and project coordinator were on site during the survey administration and circulated between classrooms to answer questions as they arose.

At the outset of the survey administration, students were asked to provide identifying information on a cover page that was detached from the survey to permit the linking of survey responses across multiple assessment waves. Prior to completing the remainder of the survey, students detached the cover page with identifying information and passed it to their teachers who placed it in an envelope and sealed it. The project director and project coordinator collected these sealed envelopes while students completed the remainder of the survey.

Study II

Design

The National Survey of Drug Use is an anonymous multi-wave survey study used to collect data on rates of substance use among school-based adolescents in Mexico. The survey was first administered in 1976 and 1986 to urban areas in 13 regions of Mexico (Medina-Mora et al., 1992). In 1991, the survey was conducted nationally by Medina-Mora and colleagues and is currently conducted biannually in Mexico City (Medina-Mora et al., 1992; Juarez et al., 1998). Data from the six northern border regions collected in 1991 were used for the current study (Medina-Mora, Villatoro, & Rojas, 1996). This sub-sample of the national data was used because it was collected in the region from which the confidential survey sample was drawn. However, for questions regarding annual and lifetime alcohol use frequency, data from the Northern regions were not available and data from the entire national sample were used. Further detail on the study procedures are outlined in Medina-Mora et al. (1992, 1996) and Villatoro et al. (1998).

Participants

The national sample from Mexico was comprised of data from 61,799 respondents. The final sample from the northern border states of Mexico was comprised of data from 13,450 respondents. Participants from the northern border states did not differ from the remaining sample. Participants were between 12 and 19 years of age with a majority of the participants (77%) being less than 15 years old and almost all (95%) being 17 years old or younger. The sample had a nearly equal proportion of females and males (51% male).

Survey Instrument

The survey is comprised mainly of items from the Monitoring the Future Survey (drug use frequency, perceived availability, social tolerance, and perception of risk) and the Center of Epidemiological Studies Depression Scale (CESD-A) (depression, suicide ideation) (Villatoro et al., 1987). The self-administered survey takes an average of 40 minutes to complete, has established reliability and validity, and has been used in most student surveys in Mexico over the past 20 years (Medina-Mora, Castro, Campillo-Serrano, & Gomez-Mont, 1981; Castro, 1987; Villatoro et al., 1998).

Procedure

Selected schools received a letter of invitation to participate in the survey. Anonymity was ensured and names of students were not included on the questionnaire. Students were informed they could refuse to participate at any time. A trained field worker administered the survey. The teacher was not in the room during administration of the survey. Seventy-eight percent of all eligible students comprising the national sample completed the survey.

Study III

Design

The Drug Use Among Adolescent Students survey is an anonymous, multi-wave cross-sectional survey of school-based adolescents in Puerto Rico (Moscoso et al., 1998). The latest survey administration occurred during the 1997-1998 school year and is the source of data used in the present study. Further detail on study procedures is outlined in Moscoso et al. (1998) and Parrilla, Moscoso, Velez, Robles, and Colon (1997).

Participants

The sample was comprised of 3,101 youth. The median age for participating middle school students was 13 and the median age for high school students who participated was 16. All students were classified as Hispanic (Puerto Rican) with a slightly higher proportion of females (53%).

Survey Instrument

The measurement instrument was designed using survey items from the Centers for Disease Control and Prevention and the Monitoring the Future survey as guides.

Procedure

Before the administration of the anonymous survey, school officials and parents of the students selected in the sample were approached to obtain their consent. Data collection was performed throughout the 1997-1998 school year by trained interviewers. Of the 5,544 students enrolled in the selected schools, 86% participated in the study.

Study IV

Design

Monitoring the Future is a national survey conducted among U.S. high school seniors since 1975 and among 8th and 10th graders since 1991. Data from 8th and 10th graders have been obtained anonymously since 1999. Data from 12th grade students were not used for the present study because they were collected using a confidential survey. Data based on the anonymous survey for 8th and 10th graders collected by the MTF in 2000 are used for the present study. Details on study procedures are available in Johnston et al. (2000).

Participants

In 2000, data from 16,700 8th grade and 14,300 10th grade students were collected. Most 8th grade (89%) and 10th grade (86%) students sampled completed the survey. The sample was comprised of students from 246 schools. There were approximately equal proportions of male and female participants. The majority of students self-identified as White (85%).

Survey Instrument

The survey is composed of items to ascertain frequency and degree of thirty-day, annual, and lifetime use of a wide variety of substances, including alcohol, marijuana, and other illicit drugs. Items asking about the perceived harmfulness and availability of drugs, parents' and friends' disapproval and attitudes toward drug use, and peer and parent drug use are also included.

Procedure

Prospective participants received an informational flyer approximately 10 days prior to the survey administration date. Local representatives generally administered the survey to 8th and 10th graders during one school class period.

Data Analysis Plan

Two-sample Z-tests of proportions were used to calculate the significance of differences in the proportions of youth reporting any lifetime use and any annual use of alcohol and marijuana between anonymous and confidential surveys. Despite some differences in response options for substance use frequency items between the anonymous and confidential surveys compared in the present study, all surveys clearly distinguished between no substance use and any substance use. Comparisons of drug use frequencies by survey format were made by gender within middle school and high school for the Mexico and Puerto Rico databases. In the U.S., comparisons of drug use frequency by survey format were made by gender for 8th and 10th grade, separately given available survey data from the Monitoring the Future Study. Given the total number of comparisons made (44), a significance value of p < .01 was adopted.

RESULTS

Mexico

Lifetime Alcohol Use. Among school-based youth in northern Mexico, there were no differences in lifetime alcohol use rates between the anonymous versus confidential survey formats for either males or females in middle school or high school (see Table 2). These non-significant differences in lifetime alcohol use rates ranged from a 1% prevalence rate difference for middle school males for the anonymous (46.7% reporting lifetime alcohol use) versus confidential (47.7%) sur-

TABLE 2. Lifetime and Annual Alcohol and Marijuana Use Rates Obtained by Anonymous and Confidential Survey Formats in Mexico by School and Gender

| | Middle School | | | | | | High School | | | | | |
| | Male | | | Female | | | Male | | | Female | | |
	A	C	D	A	C	D	A	C	D	A	C	D
Alcohol												
Lifetime	46.7	47.7	−1.0	37.1	43.5	−6.4	76.2	81.5	−5.3	67.3	68.4	−1.1
Annual	26.6	26.1	0.5	18.2	21.8	−3.6	54.2	65.0	−10.8*	41.2	48.0	−6.8*
Marijuana												
Lifetime	1.7	7.1	−5.4*	4.7	3.2	1.5	5.4	7.0	−1.6	0.8	2.0	−1.2
Annual	1.0	5.5	−4.5*	0.1	2.8	−2.7*	2.1	4.6	−2.5	0.4	1.6	−1.2*

*p < .01
A = Anonymous survey; C = Confidential Survey; D = Difference Score

veys, to a 6.4% prevalence rate difference for middle school females (i.e., 37.1% anonymous; 43.5% confidential).

Annual Alcohol Use. Annual alcohol use differed among high school males (54.2% anonymous vs. 65% confidential, z = −3.44, p < .001) and high school females (41.2% anonymous vs. 48.0% confidential, z = −2.60, p < .01). Differences in annual alcohol use rates ranged from a non-significant 0.5% prevalence rate difference for middle school males for the anonymous (26.6% reporting annual use) versus confidential (26.1%) surveys, to a significant 10.8% prevalence rate difference for high school males (i.e., 54.2% anonymous vs. 65% confidential, p < .001).

Lifetime Marijuana Use. Looking at lifetime marijuana use, only middle school males exhibited significant differences between the anonymous versus confidential survey formats (1.7% anonymous vs. 7.1% confidential, z = −6.59, p < .001) (see Table 2). Differences in lifetime marijuana use rates ranged from 1.2% prevalence rate differences for high school females for the anonymous (0.8% reporting lifetime alcohol use) versus confidential (2.0%) surveys (p > .01), to a 5.4% prevalence rate difference for middle school males (i.e., 1.7% anonymous; 7.1% confidential, p < .01).

Annual Marijuana Use. Annual marijuana use differed among middle school males (i.e., 1% anonymous; 5.5% confidential, z = −6.91, p < .001) and females (0.1% anonymous; 2.8% confidential, z = −9.06, p < .001) and high school females (0.4% anonymous; 1.6% confidential, z = −2.72, p < .01). Differences in annual marijuana use rates ranged from a 1.2% prevalence rate difference among high school females to a 4.5% prevalence rate difference among middle school males.

Puerto Rico

Lifetime Alcohol Use. Among school-based youth in Puerto Rico, there was only one difference in lifetime alcohol use rates between the anonymous versus confidential survey formats for either males or females in middle school or high school (see Table 3). Lifetime alcohol use differed among high school males (86.6% anonymous vs. 76.0% confidential, z = 3.79, p < .001). These differences in lifetime alcohol use rates ranged from 0.3% prevalence rate differences for middle school females for the anonymous (58.0% reporting lifetime alcohol use) versus confidential (58.3%) surveys (p > .01), to a 10.6% prevalence rate difference for high school males (i.e., 86.6% anonymous; 76.0% confidential).

Annual Alcohol Use. Annual alcohol use differed among high school males (75.9% anonymous vs. 60.2% confidential, z = 4.58, p < .001) and females (68.4% anonymous vs. 57.3% confidential, z = 3.54, p < .001). Annual alcohol use rates did not differ for males and females in middle school. Differences in annual alcohol use ranged from a 0.7% prevalence rate difference among middle school females to a 11.1% prevalence rate difference among high school females.

TABLE 3. Lifetime and Annual Alcohol and Marijuana Use Rates Obtained by Anonymous and Confidential Survey Formats in Puerto Rico by School and Gender

| | Middle School | | | | | | High School | | | | | |
| | Male | | | Female | | | Male | | | Female | | |
	A	C	D	A	C	D	A	C	D	A	C	D
Alcohol												
Lifetime	58.9	55.9	3.0	58.0	58.3	−0.3	86.6	76.0	10.6*	83.4	77.0	6.4
Annual	45.9	36.9	9.0	41.4	42.1	−0.7	75.9	60.2	15.7*	68.4	57.3	11.1*
Marijuana												
Lifetime	9.7	7.7	2.0	6.0	10.1	−4.1	24.8	24.0	0.8	11.2	9.4	1.8
Annual	6.7	6.2	0.5	4.0	7.7	−3.7	17.5	20.0	−2.5	7.9	6.5	1.4

*p < .01
A = Anonymous survey; C = Confidential Survey; D = Difference Score

Lifetime Marijuana Use. Looking at lifetime marijuana use, there were no significant differences between the anonymous versus confidential survey formats among males or females in middle school or high school. Differences in lifetime marijuana use rates ranged from 0.8% prevalence rate differences for high school males for the anonymous (24.8% reporting lifetime marijuana use) versus confidential (24.0%) surveys, to a 4.1% prevalence rate difference for middle school females (i.e., 6.0% anonymous; 10.1% confidential). Similarly, for annual marijuana use, there were no significant differences for any groups. Differences in annual marijuana use rates ranged from 0.5% prevalence rate differences for middle school males for the anonymous (6.7% reporting annual marijuana use) versus confidential (6.2%) surveys, to a 3.7% prevalence rate difference for middle school females (i.e., 4.0% anonymous; 7.7% confidential).

Annual Marijuana Use. For annual marijuana use, there were no significant differences for any groups. Differences in annual marijuana use rates ranged from 0.5% prevalence rate differences for middle school males for the anonymous (6.7% reporting annual marijuana use) versus confidential (6.2%) surveys, to a 3.7% prevalence rate difference for middle school females (i.e., 4.0% anonymous; 7.7% confidential).

United States

Lifetime Alcohol Use. Generally, comparisons between anonymous and confidential survey responses were non-significant (Table 4). However, a notable trend emerged for lifetime alcohol use that was significantly different in all groups (8th grade males: 51.7% anonymous vs. 67.9% confidential, $z = -4.05$, $p < .001$; 8th grade females: 51.3% anonymous vs. 63.7% confidential, $z = -2.97$, $p < .01$; 10th grade males: 71.1% anonymous vs. 82.6% confidential, $z = -2.68$, $p < .01$; 10th grade females: 71.9% anonymous vs. 88.5% confidential, $z = -3.94$, $p < .001$). Differences among prevalence rates between anonymous and confidential survey formats ranged from 11.5% (i.e., 71.1% anonymous; 82.6% confidential) to 16.6% (i.e., 71.9% anonymous; 88.5% confidential) for lifetime alcohol use.

Annual Alcohol Use. Annual alcohol use by 10th grade females differed by 14.9 percentage points (65.6% anonymous vs. 80.5% confidential, $z = -3.34$, $p < .001$). For annual alcohol use, differences ranged from 0.7 (i.e., 65.0% anonymous, 64.3% confidential) among 10th grade males ($p > .01$) to 14.9% (i.e., 65.6% anonymous, 80.5% confidential) among 10th grade females ($p < .01$). Differences among

TABLE 4. Lifetime and Annual Alcohol and Marijuana Use Rates Obtained by Anonymous and Confidential Survey Formats in the United States by School and Gender

	United States											
	8th Grade						10th Grade					
	Male			Female			Male			Female		
	A	C	D	A	C	D	A	C	D	A	C	D
Alcohol												
Lifetime	51.7	67.9	−16.2*	51.3	63.7	−12.4*	71.1	82.6	−11.5*	71.9	88.5	−16.6*
Annual	42.4	43.4	−1.0	43.6	51.4	−7.8	65.0	64.3	0.7	65.6	80.5	−14.9*
Marijuana												
Lifetime	22.2	17.6	4.6	18.1	13.7	4.4	44.2	40.9	3.3	36.3	44.2	−7.9
Annual	16.7	17.0	−0.3	14.3	13.0	1.3	36.1	34.0	2.1	28.4	34.5	−6.1

*$p < .01$
A = Anonymous survey; C = Confidential Survey; D = Difference Score

annual alcohol use ranged from a non-significant 0.7% percentage points among 10th grade males to a significant 14.9% percentage points among 10th grade females ($p < .001$).

Lifetime Marijuana Use. Looking at lifetime marijuana use among school-based youth in the United States, there were no significant differences between the anonymous versus confidential survey formats among males or females in 8th or 10th grade (see Table 4). Differences in lifetime marijuana use rates ranged from 3.3% prevalence rate differences for 10th grade males for the anonymous (44.2% reporting lifetime marijuana use) versus confidential (40.9%) surveys, to a 7.9% prevalence rate difference for 10th grade females (i.e., 36.3% anonymous; 44.2% confidential).

Annual Marijuana Use. There were no significant differences for any groups. Differences in annual marijuana use rates ranged from 0.3% prevalence rate differences for 8th grade males for the anonymous (16.7% reporting annual marijuana use) versus confidential (17.0%) surveys, to a 6.1% prevalence rate difference for 10th grade females (i.e., 28.4% anonymous; 34.5% confidential).

DISCUSSION

The findings from the present study are generally consistent with previous findings in the U.S. suggesting that in most instances, youth report comparable levels of substance use on anonymous and confidential surveys. Several response rate patterns on substance use items between anonymous and confidential survey formats emerged from the data of the present study. Only four of 44 comparisons of lifetime and annual marijuana use rates between survey formats achieved significance across the countries examined. Further, female and male school-based youth in Puerto Rico and the U.S. reported comparable lifetime and annual marijuana use rates on the anonymous and confidential surveys. Middle school students and high school females in Mexico reported higher levels of marijuana use on the confidential survey when compared to rates reported on the anonymous survey.

Compared to the findings on marijuana use rates by survey format, a greater number of differences were exhibited by school-based youth on alcohol use rates across the countries studied. For example, U.S. youth consistently reported higher lifetime alcohol prevalence rates on the confidential survey when compared to rates reported on the anonymous survey. However, annual alcohol prevalence rates reported by U.S. youth were generally comparable between survey formats. Notably, while significant differences between survey formats were achieved by U.S. youth for lifetime alcohol use, the rates of alcohol use were high across survey format as anticipated. Lifetime alcohol use rates were generally comparable between survey formats among school-based youth in Mexico and Puerto Rico with only one-of-eight comparisons achieving significance. The patterns of annual alcohol use rates between survey formats were also comparable between middle school youth in Mexico and Puerto Rico with no differences evidenced by survey format. However, high school youth in Mexico reported a higher annual alcohol use prevalence on the confidential survey while high school youth in Puerto Rico a higher annual alcohol use prevalence on the anonymous survey.

Another pattern that emerged in the present study that was not expected involved a trend toward higher not lower levels of self-reported substance use on the confidential survey format relative to the anonymous survey format. Namely, self-reported substance use prevalence rates were significantly higher for the confidential survey format for eleven of the fourteen significant differences achieved. Notably, only high school youth in Puerto Rico reported significantly lower levels of alcohol use on the confidential survey.

To some degree, each of the significant differences achieved by survey format may have occurred due to design limitations of the present study rather than survey format effects. For example, each survey used a completely different sampling frame and sampling procedure. Furthermore, varying school size and class sizes between schools studied via different survey format may have also influenced response patterns.

Despite each of these limitations, the best available anonymous survey data was used in the present study to compare against the confidential survey data collected. Still, while a variety of methodological limitations of the present study might account for the differences achieved by survey format other than the survey format itself, the potential threat to response accuracy associated with the confidential format was generally not supported in the present study. This finding is consistent with studies in the U.S. suggesting that confidential and anonymous methods produce very similar adolescent responses even on sensitive survey items (Bjarnason & Adalbjarnardottir, 2000; O'Malley et al., 2000). The need to examine whether this pattern is consistent cross-culturally is underscored by several factors. First, it is apparent that surveys of adolescent substance use in different cultures are often modeled after U.S. surveys (Medina-Mora et al., 1992; Moscoso et al., 1998). Further, data from the Current Population Survey found that in March 2000, 10% of the U.S. population was foreign-born and half (51%) were from Latin America, mostly Mexico (Lollock, 2001; Schmidley, 2001). The Center for Immigration Studies (Camarota, 2001) reports that each year approximately 400,000 legal and illegal Mexican immigrants enter the United States. Annually, approximately 95,000 of them arrived in the United States via the Del Rio Sector, which constitutes the U.S. Border Patrol area monitoring the Mexican state of Coahuila (U.S. Border Patrol, 2002), the area from which our confidential Mexico sample was drawn. Most of these Mexican immigrants attend school in the U.S. (Harriet, 1993) and complete school-based surveys.

The relative value of anonymous versus confidential survey methods involves weighing the risks and benefits of using each format along with the quality of data gathered. Institutional review boards have argued, understandably, that confidential surveys may pose a greater risk to respondents because student identities are included. However, practical experience does not support the view of greater risk. To date, no adverse events have occurred during four separate administrations of the present confidential survey across three countries. Similarly, we know of no adverse events occurring across multiple confidential surveys that have been administered to high school seniors for the Monitoring the Future study. Thus, practical experience with confidential surveys suggests that students can provide identifying data on confidential surveys without increased risk. Furthermore, Oakes (2002) outlines strategies such as encrypting identification codes and de-linking files that researchers can use to ensure confidentiality of participant survey data.

A second factor pertinent to the evaluation of the risk and benefits of confidential versus anonymous survey formats involves data integrity. On this issue, the findings of this study and related studies in the U.S. suggest that self-reported substance use rates by youth generally do not differ by confidential versus anonymous survey formats. It appears that most students are either not affected by survey format or perhaps they are indeed persuaded when trained survey proctors accurately explain that students' confidentiality will be closely guarded and protected when identifying information is provided. Whatever the reason for the lack of effects by survey format, extant findings suggest that self-reported rates of sensitive behaviors, including substance use, are valid when obtained by confidential surveys.

Anonymous surveys of youth problem behavior have been very useful at providing a snapshot of drug use rates at a given point in time. Data derived from anonymous school-based surveys have also been instrumental in developing hypotheses regarding plausible risk and protective factors associated with the onset and severity of drug use among adolescents. However, anonymous survey data have as their greatest limitation, the inability to evaluate risk factors that exhibit a causal influence on adolescent drug use and problem behavior because of the inability to link responses provided by the same students across multiple assessment waves. While multiple examples of longitudinal studies of at-risk youth exist, there has never been a cross-cultural longitudinal confidential survey study conducted to examine causal predictors of adolescent drug abuse on the scale of the Monitoring the Future study. The present study findings suggest that such a study is feasible and may be conducted without presenting elevated risk to students. Conducting such a nationwide, multi-wave, confidential survey to school-based youth would help to identify potentially malleable psychosocial risk factors contributing to the onset and severity of adolescent drug abuse which might then be addressed in existing prevention interventions.

REFERENCES

Bjarnason, T. & Adalbjarnardottir, S. (2000). Anonymity and confidentiality in school surveys on alcohol, tobacco, and cannabis use. *Journal of Drug Issues, 30*(2), 335-344.

Camarota, S.A. Immigration from Mexico: Assessing the impact on the United States. Center for Immigration Studies, 2001, *www.cis.org* (accessed August 2002).

Centers for Disease Control and Prevention *www.cdc.gov* accessed November 14, 2002.

Griffith, J., Loeb, C., & Dutil, C. (2001). 2001 Maryland Adolescent Survey: Summary of Results for Montgomery County Public Schools. Office of Shared Accountability, Montgomery County Public Schools, Rockville, Maryland.

Hallfors, D. & Iritani, B. (2002). Local and state school-based substance-use surveys. *Evaluation Review, 26*(4), 418-437.

Harriet, R. (1993). Mexican Immigrants in High Schools: Meeting Their Needs. (ERIC Document Reproduction Service No. ED 357 905). ERIC Clearinghouse on Rural Education and Small Schools. Charleston, WV.

Hibell, B., Andersson, B., Ahlstrom, S., Balakireva, O., Bjarnason, T., Kokkevi, A., & Morgan, M. (2000). The 1999 ESPAD Report: Alcohol and Other Drug Use Among Students in 30 European Countries. The Swedish Council for Information on Alcohol and Other Drugs (CAN). Publisher Modin Tryck AB, Stockholm.

Indiana Prevention Resource Center. *www.drugs.indiana.edu/drug_stats/youth.html* (accessed September 2002).

Iowa Department of Public Health. 1999 Iowa Youth Survey Report. Prepared by Iowa Consortium for Substance Abuse Research and Evaluation, University of Iowa, Iowa City. 2000

Johnston, L.D., O'Malley, P.M., & Bachman, J.G. (2002) Monitoring the Future national survey results of drug use, 1975-2001. Volume I: Secondary school students (NIH Publication No. 02-5106). Bethesda, MD: National Institute on Drug Abuse.

Johnston, L.D., O'Malley, P.M., Bachman, J.G., & Schulenberg, J. (2000) Monitoring the Future national survey results of drug use, 1975-2000. Volume I: Secondary school students (NIH Publication No. 01-4924). Bethesda, MD: National Institute on Drug Abuse.

Juarez, F., Medina-Mora, E., Berenzon, S., Villatoro, J.A., Carreno, S., Lopez, E.K., Galvan, J., & Rojas, E. (1998). Antisocial behavior: Its relation to selected sociodemographic variables and alcohol and drug use among Mexican students. *Substance Use & Misuse, 33,* 1437-1459.

Latimer, W.W., McDouall, J., Toussova, O., O'Brien, M., Floyd, L., & Vazques, M. (2004). Screening for substance abuse among school-based youth in Mexico using the Problem-Oriented Screening Instrument for Teenagers. *Substance Use and Misuse, 39,* 309-331.

Latimer, W. W., Resnick, M., & Blum, R. W. Risk and protective factors associated with adolescent alcohol use. Western Psychological Association Annual Meeting. San Jose, California, April 1996.

Latimer, W. W., Vazques, M. A., Paredes-Cortes, L. A., Zarate-Garrido, A. F., Winters, K. C., & Botzet, A. (1999, June). Drug use among school-based youth in Mexico: Predictors of problem severity and POSIT screening. In J. Anthony and G. Borges (Chairs). *Epidemiological studies on student drug involvement in Latin America.* Symposium conducted at the Sixty-First Annual Scientific Meeting of the College on Problems of Drug Dependence. Alcapulco, Mexico.

Lollock, L. U.S. Census Bureau, Current Population Reports, Series P20-534, *The Foreign-Born Population in the United States, March 2000,* U.S. Government Printing Office, Washington, DC, 2001.

McNeill, A.D., Jarvis, M.J., West, R., Russel, M.A.H., & Bryant, A. Saliva cotine as an indicator of cigarette smoking in adolescents. *British Journal of Addictions* 1987, 82, 1355-1360.

Medina-Mora, M.E., Castro, S., Campillo-Serrano, C., & Gomez-Mont, F.A. (1981). Validity and reliability of a high school drug use questionnaire among Mexican students. *Bulletin on Narcotics, 33* (4), 67-76.

Medina-Mora, M.E., Rojas, E., Galvan, J., Juarez, F., Berenzon, S., Carreno, S., Villatoro, J., Lopez, E., Ortiz, E., & Olmedo, R. (December, 1992). Drug use among Mexican student youth. *CEWG*, 483-494.

Medina-Mora, M. E., Villatoro, J., & Rojas, E. (1996). Drug use among students in Mexico's northern border states. *CEWG*, 367-379.

Moscoso, M. R., Parrilla, I., Robles, R. R., Colon, H. M., & Garcia, M. (1998). El uso de drogas en los escolares puertorriquenos. *Consulta Juvenil IV*, 1997-98.

Oakes, J.M. (2002). Risks and wrongs in social science research: An evaluator's guide to the IRB. *Evaluation Review, 26*(5), 443-479.

O'Brien, M.S. & Latimer, W. W. (2002, August). Adolescent Substance Use Disorders in Mexico, Puerto Rico, and the United States, In W. W. Latimer (Chair), *Multi-ethnic and multi-national examination of adolescent drug abuse risks and diagnosis.* Symposium conducted at the meeting of the 2002 American Psychological Association Annual Convention, Chicago, Illinois.

Ohio Department of Alcohol and Drug Addiction Services & Ohio Department of Education. *www2.state.oh.us/ada/news.html* (accessed November 2002).

O'Malley, P.M., Johnston, L.D., Bachman, J.G., & Schulenber, J. (2000). A comparison of confidential versus anonymous survey procedures: Effects on reporting of drug use and related attitudes and beliefs in a national study of students. *Journal of Drug Issues, 30*(1), 35-54.

Parrilla, I.C., Moscoso, M.R., Velez, M., Robles, R.R., & Colon, H.M. (1997). Internal and external environment of the Puerto Rican adolescents in the use of alcohol, drugs and violence. *Bol Asoc Med P R, 89*(7-9), 146-149.

Pride Surveys. *www.pridesurveys.com* (accessed November 2002).

Rhode Island Department of Health. The 1998 Rhode Island Adolescent Substance Abuse Survey: Report for Statewide Results. Office of Health Statistics, Rhode Island Department of Health. Prepared by ORC Macro, Burlington, Vermont.

Schmidley, A.D. U.S. Census Bureau, Current Population Reports, Series P23-206, *Profile of the Foreign-Born Population in the United States: 2000*, U.S. Government Printing Office, Washington, DC, 2001.

U.S. Border Patrol Del Rio Sector expanding boat patrol to reduce flow of illegal immigrants. United States Department of Justice, 2002, *www.ins.usdoj.gov* (accessed August 2002).

Villatoro, J.A., Medina-Mora, E., Juarez, F., Rojas, E., Carreno, S., & Berenzon, S. (1998). Drug use pathways among high school students of Mexico. *Addiction, 93,* 1577-1588.

Wallisch, L.S. & Liu, L.Y. (1999). 1998 Texas School Survey of Substance Use Among Students: Grades 4-6. Texas Commission on Alcohol and Drug Abuse. Austin, TX. *www.tcada.state.tx.us* (accessed November 2002).

Winters, K. C., Latimer, W. W., & Stinchfield, R. D. Adolescent treatment. *In Source book on substance abuse: Etiology, epidemiology, assessment, and treatment*; Ott, P. J., Tarter, R. E., Ammerman, R. T., Eds.; Allyn and Bacon: New York, 1999; 350-361.

Winters, K.C. & Henly, G.A. *Adolescent Diagnostic Interview and Manual*. Los Angeles: Western Psychological Services. 1993

Winters, K.C. & Henly, G.A. *Personal Experience Inventory and Manual*. Los Angeles: Western Psychological Services. 1989

doi:10.1300/J029v16n01_06

Gender Differences
in Measuring Adolescent Drug Abuse
and Related Psychosocial Factors

Andria M. Botzet
Ken C. Winters
Randy Stinchfield

SUMMARY. Although gender issues have been addressed in clinical drug abuse literature, very little research has focused on gender differences in terms of the psychometric properties of assessment instruments. If boys and girls interpret instruments differently, the accuracy of clinical evaluation, referral, and treatment decisions based on these measures may be compromised. The current study examines this issue within the context of one instrument, the Personal Experience Inventory (PEI). The PEI is a multi-scale, self-administered questionnaire that has been used in various descriptive and treatment studies of adolescent drug abusers. We examine gender-specific psychometric properties of the PEI based on a drug-abusing sample of adolescents (n of boys = 1,322; n of girls = 822). The results indicate that reliability and validity evidence, as well as

Andria M. Botzet, MA, Ken C. Winters, PhD, and Randy Stinchfield, PhD, are affiliated with the Department of Psychiatry, University of Minnesota.

Address correspondence to: Andria M. Botzet, MA, Department of Psychiatry, University of Minnesota, F282/2A West, 2450 Riverside Avenue, Minneapolis, MN 55454 (E-mail: botze003@umn.edu).

Support for this manuscript was provided from NIDA grants DA05104 and K02 DA15347.

[Haworth co-indexing entry note]: "Gender Differences in Measuring Adolescent Drug Abuse and Related Psychosocial Factors." Botzet, Andria M., Ken C. Winters, and Randy Stinchfield. Co-published simultaneously in *Journal of Child & Adolescent Substance Abuse* (The Haworth Press, Inc.) Vol. 16, No. 1, 2006, pp. 91-108; and: *Adolescent Substance Abuse: New Frontiers in Assessment* (ed: Ken C. Winters) The Haworth Press, Inc., 2006, pp. 91-108. Single or multiple copies of this article are available for a fee from The Haworth Document Delivery Service [1-800-HAWORTH, 9:00 a.m. - 5:00 p.m. (EST). E-mail address: docdelivery@haworthpress.com].

doi:10.1300/J029v16n01_07

factor structure data, are generally comparable for both genders. However, differences did arise in rates of elevation on the distortion scales. Limitations of the present study and future research needs are discussed. doi:10.1300/J029v16n01_07 *[Article copies available for a fee from The Haworth Document Delivery Service: 1-800-HAWORTH. E-mail address: <docdelivery@haworthpress.com> Website: <http://www.HaworthPress.com> © 2006 by The Haworth Press, Inc. All rights reserved.]*

KEYWORDS. Gender differences, assessment, PEI, drug abuse, adolescents

Several clinical and epidemiological studies have addressed gender issues in adolescent drug abuse research. Prevalence studies have predominantly found that boys are at a greater risk for alcohol and other drug abuse (Kahler, Read, Wood, & Palfai, 2003), and that boys are more likely to try illicit drugs and more likely to use them more frequently than girls (Johnston, O'Malley, Bachman, & Schulenberg, 2005). According to the 2005 Monitoring the Future Study, boys also report much higher rates of smokeless tobacco, steroid use, and heavy drinking. However, cigarette use is roughly the same across genders (Johnston et al., 2005). A recent national report of drug use among Americans indicated that adolescent boys reported higher rates on nearly every drug use variable, including early onset of drug use, binge drinking, illicit drug use, and substance use disorders (Substance Abuse and Mental Health Services Administration, 2005).

Clinical studies have revealed gender differences and similarities with respect to determinants of gender differences, including social and cultural environment, psychological and physical health factors, and coping mechanisms. Opland, Winters, and Stinchfield (1995) found that girls tend to utilize drug use as a coping mechanism for stress, whereas boys tend to use drugs for the pleasurable effects. A cross-sectional study of drug-abusing youth assessed in clinical settings (Winters, Stinchfield, & Henly, 1993) found that scales measuring delinquency and peer drug involvement were most highly correlated with overall drug use involvement in both girls and boys. However, girls tended to have higher associations between drug involvement and psychological distress compared to boys. A study by Hsieh and Hollister (2004) found that female subjects who were entering a substance abuse treatment program exhibited more severe psychological difficulties, poorer self-image, increased family problems, and more exposure to sexual abuse than did their male counterparts. Meanwhile, boys in the same study exhibited higher rates of school and legal problems as compared to the girls. Dakof, Tejeda, and Liddle (2000) found similar results in their clinical sample, namely, that drug-abusing girls exhibited much higher levels of internalizing symptoms and higher levels of family dysfunction, even though they used drugs just as extensively as the boys.

Of importance to this literature is the relative impact of the psychometric soundness of the instruments used to infer findings related to gender. If measures are biased by gender, the interpretation of study results may be potentially jeopardized. For example, males and females may differ on their report of feelings and emotions, which could influence a measure that depends on emotive-related issues. Also, self-report may vary by gender; one gender may be more likely to under-report or over-report certain aspects of drug involvement. Several reviews are available on the state of the adolescent drug abuse assessment field (e.g., Leccese & Waldron, 1994; Winters, 2003), and this literature concludes that, as a group, the clinical instruments and measures used within this field have generally favorable psychometric properties. However, there has been virtually no focus on the relative psychometric evidence of these instruments by gender.

This paper addresses the issue of gender differences in the measurement of drug abuse severity and related psychosocial factors by focusing on a single instrument, the Personal Experience Inventory (PEI: Winters & Henly, 1989). The PEI is a relevant tool to address gender-specific issues because it has been widely cited in the literature (Rahdert, 1991; Weinberg et al., 1998), a large clinical database of girls and boys now exists, and its multidimensionality allows for both drug abuse and psychosocial scales to be examined. Previous publications of the PEI's psychometric properties have not fully addressed the issue of gender. The PEI manual only reports one set of psychometric data as a function of gender: scale internal consistency (Winters & Henly, 1989). These data show comparable coefficient alphas for both boys and girls. Another study by Winters, Latimer, Stinchfield, and Henly (1999) found that correlations between the Psychosocial scales and Drug Use Frequency (DUF) scales on the PEI were similar among age and gender groups. That study also found that the Psychological Disturbance, Peer Chemical Environment, Deviant Behavior, and Negative Self-Image scales were most predictive of DUF for both genders (Winters et al.,

1999). Other publications on the psychometrics of the PEI have not reported gender specific data, most certainly because the small sample sizes in these studies precluded such comparisons (e.g., Guthmann & Brenna, 1990; Cady, Winters, Jordan, Solberg, & Stinchfield, 1996).

The present study capitalizes on a large PEI database that has been built for over eight years. We report a range of reliability and validity evidence as a function of gender and age (younger = 12-15 years old; older = 16-18 years old) subgroups. Our intent was to additionally sub-divide the subjects into ethnic groups as a function of gender and age. However, because the database has very small sample sizes of younger and older girls among the non-white ethnic groups (range 0.5%-6% for Hispanic, African American, Asian, and American Indian groups), we limited this study to White youth. These adjustments led to a final sample size of 2,144 adolescents meeting study criteria (described below). We describe psychometric evidence pertaining to internal reliability, test-retest reliability, convergent validity, factor structure, and elevations on the response distortion scales. We are not proposing any specific hypotheses, given that this investigation is descriptive in nature and the extant literature does not provide any guidance in this light.

METHOD

Measure

The PEI was developed to address the multitude of behaviors and psychosocial factors believed to be directly related to drug involvement. Its 278 items are primarily broken down into two sections (Problem Severity and Psychosocial); additional items measure drug use frequency and response distortion tendencies.

Part 1: Problem Severity Scales. This section of the PEI consists of a core set of five drug abuse problem severity scales, called the Basic Scales, as well as a secondary set of problem severity scales, the Clinical Scales. The Basic Scales cover a broad range of adolescent drug involvement, including perceived social and psychological benefits, negative social and personal consequences, polydrug use, and loss of control. They were developed from a combination of rational and empirical procedures, such as literature reviews, consultation with experts, and factor analyses (see Henly & Winters, 1988, for details). Four of these five scales consist of 8-11 items each, with a 4-point response option set (never, once or twice, sometimes, often) for each item. The remaining Basic Scale, the Personal Involvement with Chemicals Scale (PICS), consists of 29 items. The PICS was purposely created with a larger number of items than the other scales with the intent that it would adequately measure a general drug abuse severity construct and would also measure outlier patterns of drug use experiences (Henly & Winters, 1988).

The five Clinical Scales, which consist of some redundant items assigned to the PICS, focus on drug abuse content intended to be particularly relevant to clinical referral and treatment issues (e.g., signs of dependence; additional attributions of use). However, these scales do not add any substantial variance beyond the PICS (Henly & Winters, 1988). Given the redundancy of these scales, the analysis for this paper focused primarily on the set of Basic Scales.

Part 2: Psychosocial Scales. The second section of the PEI is comprised of 12 Psychosocial Scales that measure risk factors believed to be related to the onset and maintenance of youth drug involvement (Henly & Winters, 1989). Eight of these scales concentrate on Personal Adjustment, such as Negative Self-Image and Social Isolation, while the remaining four scales relate to Environmental Risk, including Peer Chemical Use and Family Pathology, among others. Items in each of these scales are measured on either a 4-point response option structure (strongly agree, agree, disagree, strongly disagree) or a 3-point response option format (never, once or twice, sometimes), and the number of items per scale ranges from 4-12. Development of these scales began with 20 *a priori* scales identified from existing literature. Scales with acceptable levels of reliability (alpha > .70) were retained, along with those showing independence (proportion of unique, reliable variance > .25). Redundant scales were discarded, and items were pruned from their respective scales if they had a high correlation with the Marlowe-Crowne Desirability Scale (Crowne & Marlowe, 1960). The result of these reductions was the 12 scales that encompass the Psychosocial section of the PEI.

Additional Content. Both parts of the PEI (Problem Severity and Psychosocial) include supplemental items that measure response distortion. Two separate but parallel sets of response distortion items were created to accommodate users of the PEI who may only administer one of the sections. The response distortion items cover Infrequency ("faking bad," inattention, random responses) and Defensiveness ("faking good"). The Infrequency scales contain 7 items in Part 1 and 11 items in Part 2; these scales reflect very low rates of endorsement as they refer to extremely unlikely behaviors and attitudes. Defensiveness items (11 and 12 items, in Part 1 and Part 2, respectively) are used to measure defensiveness or social desirability, based on the Marlowe-Crowne Social Desirability Scale (Crowne & Marlowe, 1960). Cases that report an elevated level (T-score $\geq$ 70) on these scales may reflect that an accurate portrait of the respondent's behaviors and attitudes is not being reported. For the present analyses, cases were removed if such an elevation occurred for any of the four response distortion scales (the exception to this is the analysis we conducted on response distortion rates by gender).

Finally, there is a set of Drug Use Frequency (DUF) items located in Part I that measures the frequency of alcohol and other drug use during the following time points: *past 3-months, prior year* and *lifetime*. DUF items are consistent with standard drug use frequency items from the National Institute of Health annual survey of drug use behavior among American high school students (Johnston, O'Malley, & Bachman, 2001). Respondents report their drug use frequency during each time point using a categorical 7-point response option (never, once or twice, 3-5 times, 5-9 times, 10-19 times, 20-39 times, 40 or more times) for each of 12 drug categories. For purposes of this study, we have created an aggregate of all 12 drug categories for each of the *lifetime* and *prior year* categories. Thus, those who have never used any type of drug would score a 7, while those who report use of every drug "40 or more times" would score 84.

Psychometrics. Previous publications on the PEI have reported a range of psychometric properties. Internal consistency reliability data are favorable; alphas are .75 or higher (Winters & Henly, 1989). Test-retest reliability measures reveal stability correlations ranging from .40-.92 for one-week retest, and .44-.85 for one-month retest across all scales (Guthmann & Brenna, 1990; Henly & Winters, 1988; Jainchill, Yagelka, Hawke, & De Leon, 1999). Concurrent validity tests for the Problem Severity scales show that scale coefficients generally exceeded .50 when the PEI was compared to parallel client measures and counselor ratings of drug abuse severity (Winters, Stinchfield, & Henly, 1996). Construct validity evidence is indicated by significant between-group differences on Problem Severity and Psychosocial scales among clinical samples (school, juvenile detention, and drug abuse treatment samples) and non-clinical samples (no referrals to primary treatment, outpatient treatment, or residential treatment). Construct validity is generally stronger for the Problem Severity scales compared to the Psychosocial scales (Winters & Henly, 1989; Henly & Winters,

1988; Henly & Winters, 1989). Also, a recent analysis of drug-clinic referred boys indicates that the PEI's reliability, validity and factor structure are comparable across four ethnic groups (African American, American Indian, Hispanic, and White) (Winters, Latimer, Stinchfield, & Egan, 2005).

Participants

Data for this analysis is based on PEI responses from 2,144 white participants in eight different adolescent drug abuse assessment and/or treatment programs throughout Minnesota and Canada over an 8-year period (1994-2002). These programs supplied PEI scores for purposes of assessment research, as part of a drug clinic database that provides sociodemographic and clinical data. Programs varied in type (assessment only, private, or public), modality (residential or outpatient), and intensity (duration of contact). Participating programs were required to adhere to rigorous administration procedures, as outlined in the PEI manual, and then send completed PEI test booklets to the principal investigator at the University of Minnesota. Two clinics, however, only contributed .5% or less of the sample and were thus eliminated from the analyses to minimize a recruitment cohort effect. The remaining programs contributed between 5% and 40% of the sample.

Youth had to meet the following criteria in order to be eligible for the present study: (1) they were specifically referred for an intake assessment due to suspected drug use; (2) they were able to read English at a 5th grade level or greater, as screened by procedures in the PEI manual; (3) they were not intoxicated or suffering from withdrawal symptoms; (4) they were not acutely psychotic or mentally impaired at the time of testing; (5) they identified themselves ethnically as White, as recorded on their PEI score sheet/item booklet; and (6) they did not meet response distortion or unscorable test criteria. With respect to the last inclusion criterion, cases were omitted if any of the four response distortion scales were elevated (T-score $\geq$ 70) or if there were too many unscorable or omitted responses ($\geq$ 20% of items in scale). Invalid responses accounted for 12.5% of cases among boys and 8.4% of cases among girls in this sample. The sample of 2,144 used in the analyses (except test-retest) represents the cases that met all inclusion criteria, including the absence of any elevations on the response distortion scales and absence of meeting unscoreable test criteria. The analysis of response distortion rates focused on those cases that had elevations on one or more of the response distortion scales. Due to limitations in resources, test-retest data was collected as part of the PEI database for only a subset of the sample. After applying study criteria, the sample available for test-retest analysis were 570 youth (37.7% girls; 37.0% younger age group).

Procedure

Subjects who met the criteria listed above were asked to voluntarily participate in an assessment research study during the course of their intake process at a participating program. The youth who were interested signed an assent form; parental consent was then sought. For youth over the age of 17, signed parental consent was not required. Following the consent process, either the research staff (for local treatment programs) or the program staff (for non-local treatment sites) administered the PEI within 3 days of intake to the program. All staff members were trained in administering the PEI through use of the manual.

For all but three of the treatment sites, program staff did not have access to individual PEI results. At the three exception sites, program staff computed their own PEI score reports because they had purchased the computer-scoring software. For non-local programs, youth filled out the paper-pencil PEI questionnaires and the completed product was mailed to U of M research staff in a sealed envelope. Consent forms were appropriately adjusted to reflect these deviations in confidentiality.

RESULTS

A demographic summary of the sample is provided in Table 1. As shown, the sample sizes of each gender group are acceptable for purposes of statistical analysis. Average age of girls was 15.5 years (sd = 1.3) and 16.0 years (sd = 1.2) for boys ($t = 9.81, p < .001$). Given that age has been shown to be related to PEI scale scores (Winters & Henly, 1989), we decided to organize the psychometric tests by gender-age subgroups (younger = ages 12-15 years; older = 16-18 years). Therefore, our group comparisons were structured according to the following pairwise comparisons (% of total sample in parentheses): Younger Boys (19.5%) versus Younger Girls (17.9%) (YB vs YG), and Older Boys (42.2%) versus Older Girls (20.5%) (OB vs OG).

TABLE 1. Demographic Characteristics of the Drug Clinic Sample (n = 2,144) by Age and Gender Group

Variable	Younger Group (ages 12-15)		Older Group (ages 16-18)	
	Boys (n = 418)	Girls (n = 383)	Boys (n = 904)	Girls (n = 439)
% of total sample	19.5	17.9	42.2	20.5
% of gender	31.6	46.6	68.4	53.4
% of age group	52.2	47.8	67.3	32.7
% Used alcohol, prior year[a]	95.3	96.7	97.7	96.7
% Used marijuana, prior year[b]	86.1	82.0	87.4	82.5
% History of psychiatric problems	21.3	35.8	20.6	34.2
% History of family drug abuse	58.9	64.0	52.4	55.6

Note. Drug use variables, psychiatric history, and family history are based on results from the Personal Experience Inventory (Winters & Henly, 1989).
[a] 64 cases did not report alcohol use during the past year.
[b] 67 cases did not report marijuana use during the past year.

Reliability

Internal Consistency. This measure of internal reliability is intended to quantify the similarity between the items in a given scale, suggesting that the items are measuring one "true" construct. Generally, a Cronbach coefficient alpha of .70 or higher is considered optimal for research purposes. Coefficient alpha data in this sample showed a high level of reliability, with most scales falling in the range of .80-.90 (range .68-.97; median = .85) (see Table 2). All pairwise groups (YB vs YG and OB vs OG) were fairly matched on alpha levels. The Basic Scales generally produced the highest alphas, especially the PICS scale (Personal Involvement with Chemicals), which had alphas at .96-.97 for both boys and girls. The lowest alphas were consistently found among the Psychosocial scales. One scale showed a notable group difference: Social Isolation. On this scale, the YB fell just below the optimal .70 alpha cutoff (YB = .63), whereas the alpha for the YG was above the cutoff (.78).

Temporal Stability. Temporal stability indicates an instrument's ability to measure the same construct over a given period of time. Participants complete the same instrument twice, with the two assessments separated by time. Data from the two time-points are then correlated,

TABLE 2. Internal Consistency (Coefficient Alpha) Reliability Estimates of PEI Scales as a Function of Age and Gender Groups

PEI Scales	Younger Group (ages 12-15)		Older Group (ages 16-18)	
	Boys (n = 418)	Girls (n = 383)	Boys (n = 904)	Girls (n = 439)
Basic Problem Severity				
Personal Involvement	.97	.96	.97	.97
Effects from Drug Use	.89	.90	.89	.90
Social Benefits	.86	.84	.88	.89
Personal Consequences	.90	.82	.89	.87
Polydrug Use	.82	.78	.86	.83
Psychosocial				
Negative Self-Image	81	.87	.85	.90
Psychological Disturbance	.82	.81	.80	.82
Social Isolation	.63	.78	.70	.77
Uncontrolled	.85	.90	.85	.86
Rejecting Convention	.74	.79	.75	.76
Deviant Behavior	.83	.79	.83	.78
Absence of Goals	.81	.86	.80	.83
Spiritual Isolation	.86	.90	.88	.88
Peer Chemical Use	.82	.86	.84	.86
Sibling Chemical Use	.84	.85	.85	.84
Family Pathology	.78	.79	.80	.81
Family Estrangement	.82	.87	.83	.87

with the expectation that the two testings will correlate highly ($\geq .70$) in a reliable instrument. In this study, the retest interval was one week after the first testing. Sample sizes for this analysis were as follows: YB = 110; YG = 101; OB = 245; OG = 114. The one-week test-retest data revealed that scale stability coefficients, while somewhat variable, were comparable across groups. All correlations were significant at $p < .01$, and no between-group differences were significant. Estimates of temporal stability for the Basic Scales ranged from .70 to .91, with a median of .74; stability estimates for the Psychosocial Scales were generally lower and more variable compared to the Basic Scales; they ranged from .51 to .89, with a median of .71. The Psychosocial Scales that consistently showed the lowest temporal stability were Psychological Disturbance (.51-.52), Uncontrolled (.53-.57), and Negative Self-Image (.54-.55). The Psychosocial Scales with the highest temporal stability coefficients were Sibling Chemical Use (.84-.86) and Deviant Behavior (.89-.90).

Validity

Convergent Validity. This form of validity measures the similarity between the target construct and an alternate measure of the construct. A higher correlation between the two measures is interpreted as stronger evidence of validity for the target measure; a moderate correlation is deemed to be .30 or greater, whereas a high correlation is considered to be .60 or greater. Because the Basic Scales of the PEI intend to measure problem severity among adolescent drug use behavior, they should be positively associated with drug use frequency measures for this analysis. Tables 3 (prior year drug use) and 4 (lifetime drug use) show the correlations of the PEI scales by drug use frequency according to groups. Both genders and age groups showed moderate to high correlations (all correlations exceeded .40). In general, Basic Scales–Lifetime DUF correlations were higher than Basic Scales–Prior Year DUF correlations. Convergent validity coefficients did not significantly differ be-

TABLE 3. Correlations of PEI Scales and Aggregate Measure of Prior Year Drug Use Frequency as a Function of Age and Gender Groups

PEI Scales	Younger Group (ages 12-15)				Older Group (ages 16-18)			
	Boys (n = 418)	Girls (n = 383)	z^a	p	Boys (n = 904)	Girls (n = 439)	z^a	p
Basic Problem Severity								
Personal Involvement	.67	.68	−.26	.79	.68	.63	1.47	.14
Effects from Drug Use	.55	.53	−.96	.34	.55	.47	1.80	.07
Social Benefits	.47	.42	.89	.37	.44	.40	.69	.49
Personal Consequences	.64	.60	.93	.35	.61	.61	0	1.00
Polydrug Use	.84	.85	−.50	.62	.81	.81	0	1.00
Psychosocial								
Negative Self-Image	.22	.29	−1.07	.28	.24	.25	−.17	.87
Psychological Disturbance	.40	.32	1.31	.19	.30	.23	1.27	.20
Social Isolation	.07	.23	−2.34	.02	.15	.19	−.68	.50
Uncontrolled	.37	.36	.16	.87	.31	.21	1.72	.09
Rejecting Convention	.19	.31	−1.84	.07	.22	.27	−.88	.38
Deviant Behavior	.44	.47	−.54	.59	.44	.43	.20	.84
Absence of Goals	.24	.28	−.61	.54	.21	.22	−.18	.86
Spiritual Isolation	−.12	.10	−3.16	.00	−.02	.04	−1.00	.32
Peer Chemical Use	.41	.43	−.34	.73	.50	.43	1.48	.14
Sibling Chemical Use	.19	.15	.59	.56	.21	.17	.68	.50
Family Pathology	.23	.12	1.61	.11	.19	.13	1.02	.31
Family Estrangement	.15	.28	−1.96	.05	.15	.07	1.35	.18

[a] Refers to the *z* transformation testing for differences in the correlations.

TABLE 4. Correlations of PEI Scales and Aggregate Lifetime Drug Use Frequency as a Function of Age and Gender Groups

PEI Scales	Younger Group (ages 12-15)				Older Group (ages 16-18)			
	Boys (n = 418)	Girls (n = 383)	z^a	p	Boys (n = 904)	Girls (n = 439)	z^a	p
Basic Problem Severity								
Personal Involvement	.65	.64	.24	.81	.67	.55	3.22	.00
Effects from Drug Use	.52	.51	.19	.85	.56	.40	3.48	.00
Social Benefits	.45	.40	.87	.38	.49	.40	1.92	.05
Personal Consequences	.61	.58	.67	.50	.62	.55	1.78	.08
Polydrug Use	.83	.86	−1.50	.13	.86	.80	3.23	.00
Psychosocial								
Negative Self-Image	.20	.25	−.74	.46	.25	.17	1.38	.17
Psychological Disturbance	.36	.30	.96	.34	.32	.17	2.67	.01
Social Isolation	.07	.22	−2.20	.03	.14	.17	−.52	.60
Uncontrolled	.34	.34	0	1.00	.32	.15	3.02	.00
Rejecting Convention	.20	.30	−1.53	.13	.18	.24	−1.05	.29
Deviant Behavior	.44	.48	−.73	.47	.51	.46	1.10	.27
Absence of Goals	.23	.23	0	1.00	.18	.21	−.52	.60
Spiritual Isolation	−.09	.12	−3.01	.00	−.05	.04	−1.50	.13
Peer Chemical Use	.40	.41	−.17	.87	.45	.35	2.03	.04
Sibling Chemical Use	.15	.17	−.30	.76	.22	.14	1.38	.17
Family Pathology	.20	.16	.60	.55	.20	.15	.87	.38
Family Estrangement	.14	.27	−1.94	.05	.13	.06	1.18	.24

[a]Refers to the *z* transformation testing for differences in the correlations.

tween groups for the Basic Scales–Prior Year DUF data. However, 4 of the 5 correlations for the Basic Scales–Lifetime DUF showed statistically significantly higher coefficients for the OB group compared to the OG group.

Discriminant Validity. Contrary to the goals of convergent validity, discriminant validity attempts to show that the target construct is dissimilar to a different construct. In this situation, a lower correlation would indicate the dissimilarities desired for a stronger measure of validity. Although the Psychosocial Risk scales of the PEI are expected to have an association with drug use frequency (Hawkins, Catalano, & Miller, 1992; Henly & Winters, 1989), they are not expected to be related to drug use frequency at the same high magnitude as observed with the Basic Scales. Subsequently, we observed correlations of drug use frequency with the Psychosocial Risk scales that were quite low (see lower portions of Table 3 and 4). No correlations exceeded .50 for Prior Year DUF, and no correlations exceeded .48 for Lifetime DUF. Seventy percent and 73% of the correlations were at or below .30 for Prior Year and Lifetime DUF data, respectively. There was a noteworthy group difference: YG had higher correlations than YB for both sets of DUF correlations for Social Isolation, Spiritual Isolation and Family Estrangement. Also, the Psychosocial scales that had the highest correlations with lifetime and prior year DUF were the Peer Chemical Use scale and the Deviant Behavior scale. These moderate correlations are not surprising, given the relationships among deviant behavior and peer drug use with one's own drug involvement (Latimer, Winters, Stinchfield, & Traver, 2000; Raniseski & Sigelman, 1992). Spiritual Isolation consistently had the lowest correlations across all groups ($-.12$ to .12).

Factor Analysis. A Principal Component Analysis (PCA) was conducted to explore if the factor structure of the PEI is similar for boys and girls (see Table 5). PCA is a statistical technique that correlates common factors in a given set, condensing a large set of items into smaller, more similar constructs. For the sake of parsimony, the PCA was conducted for each gender group without consideration of age subgroups. Results revealed that three factors were identified for boys and girls and that loadings on them were quite similar for both genders. The first component for boys and girls consisted of the 5 Basic Scales, Deviant Behavior, Peer Chemical Environment, and Sibling Chemical Use. The Uncontrolled scale was an additional scale for the first component for boys. Common scales for both genders in the second factor were Negative Self-image, Family Estrangement, Psychological Disturbance, Family Pathology, and Social Isolation. The Uncontrolled scale also fell into the second component for girls, and the boys' second component also included Absence of Goals. The third component consisted of Rejecting Convention and Spiritual Isolation for girls and boys; Absence of Goals was also assigned to this third factor for girls.

Response Distortion. Elevated responses on at least one response distortion scale occurred in 264 cases (11% of the total sample; 12.5% among boys and 8.4% among girls). The group comparison (see Table 6) revealed that a significantly greater percentage of YB's generated elevated scores on three of the four response distortion scales compared to YG's (χ^2 range, 4.4-11.5). Also, the OB group had significantly higher elevation rates than the OG group on both Infrequency scales ($\chi^2 = 20.2$ and 11.7, respectively). There were no significant differences between groups for one scale, Defensiveness-2.

TABLE 5. Principal Component Factor Analysis of PEI Scales for Boys and Girls

Pattern Matrix–Boys				Pattern Matrix–Girls			
	Factor				Factor		
	1	2	3		1	2	3
Personal Involvement with Chemicals	.920	.018	−.063	Personal Involvement with Chemicals	.878	.126	−.158
Personal Consequences of Drug Use	.889	.031	−.054	Personal Consequences of Drug Use	.868	.008	−.084
Polydrug Use	.845	−.064	−.001	Polydrug Use	.814	−.055	.054
Peer Chemical Environment	.746	−.103	.175	Deviant Behavior	.691	−.096	.266
Deviant Behavior	.734	−.126	.165	Effects from Drug Use	.658	.368	−.264
Effects from Drug Use	.730	.244	−.200	Social Benefits of Drug Use	.639	.277	.300
Social Benefits of Drug Use	.713	.106	−.155	Peer Chemical Environment	.609	.052	.142
Uncontrolled	.422	.392	.158	Sibling Chemical Use	.257	−.066	.220
Sibling Chemical Use	.299	.056	.001	Negative Self-Image	.083	.813	−.167
Negative Self-Image	.131	.750	−.077	Psychological Disturbance	.140	.755	−.219
Family Estrangement	−.116	.712	.224	Family Estrangement	−.149	.689	.259
Psychological Disturbance	.239	.667	−.233	Social Isolation	−.023	.680	.177
Family Pathology	.018	.587	−.151	Uncontrolled	.305	.509	.108
Social Isolation	−.030	.580	.378	Family Pathology	.018	.470	.018
Absence of Goals	.066	.486	.455	Rejecting Convention	.205	.195	.672
Rejecting Convention	.206	.131	.744	Spiritual Isolation	−.061	.088	.667
Spiritual Isolation	−.050	−.083	.691	Absence of Goals	.057	.486	.489

Note: Age groups within each gender are collapsed for this analysis.

DISCUSSION

The purpose of this study was to examine gender differences within the context of psychometric properties of the PEI. The study produced three major findings. First, the reliability and validity of the PEI was similar for boys and girls, regardless of age group. This pattern of results was observed for both the Problem Severity and Psychosocial Risk scales across a range of psychometric tests. Based on these data, the PEI does not appear to show differential psychometric properties as a function of gender. It should be noted, however, that our convergent and discriminant validity analyses were limited to only one criterion

TABLE 6. Prevalence (%) of Elevations on the PEI Response Distortion Scales as a Function of Age and Gender Groups

Group	Younger Group (ages 12-15)			Older Group (ages 16-18)		
	Boys (n = 418) %	Girls (n = 383) %	χ^2	Boys (n = 904) %	Girls (n = 439) %	χ^2
Infrequency −1	4.4	2.1	4.38*	5.6	0.9	20.21 ***
Infrequency −2	9.5	4.1	11.52 ***	5.1	1.5	11.72 ***
Defensiveness −1	7.9	4.4	5.09*	6.2	4.7	1.37
Defensiveness −2	3.5	2.8	.35	5.2	4.4	.40

Notes. The Infrequency scales measure "faking-bad" and inattention, and the Defensiveness scales measure "faking-good." Figures do not represent mutually exclusive groups. These cases were not included in the psychometric analyses.

* $p < .05$; *** $p < .001$

variable–drug use frequency. An expanded list of criterion variables (e.g., concurrent diagnoses, referral decisions) would be useful to include in future research.

The second major finding is that the PCA suggests that the factor structure of the PEI is generally similar for boys and girls. The noteworthy exception pertains to the Uncontrolled scale. This scale measures behaviors that reflect impulsivity and oppositional traits (e.g., "I get angry and lose my temper"; "I do the opposite of what people tell me, just to make them mad"; "People complain that I don't listen to them"). For boys, the Uncontrolled scale loaded more heavily on the first factor which included the BASIC problem severity scales, Peer Chemical Environment and Deviant Behavior. This finding is consistent with other research that links Oppositional Defiant Disorder with higher levels of drug abuse, especially among boys (see Barkley, Fischer, Edelbrock, & Smallish, 1990; Biederman, Wilens, Mick & Faraone, 1997). For girls, the Uncontrolled scale loaded on the second component, along with scales such as Negative Self-Image, Social Isolation, and Family Estrangement. This finding falls in line with Hsieh and Hollister's (1994) data that girls who abuse drugs have a poorer self-image than boys.

A third major conclusion of this study conveys that a higher percentage of boys revealed elevations on nearly all of the PEI response distortion scales compared to girls. This finding raises the issue that boys in general may give more invalid self-reports than girls. It is tempting to draw a causal connection between our finding that boys score higher on the Deviant Behavior scale (Henly & Winters, 1989) and reveal elevated rates of response distortion compared to girls. Indeed, a post-hoc test revealed such a pattern. We compared invalid responding boys and girls (defined by an elevation on any distortion scale) on the Deviant Behavior scale. "Invalid" boys scored significantly higher than "invalid" girls on this scale (M boys = 17.6; M girls = 15.2; $t = 4.4$, $p < .00$). Nonetheless, very little research has thus far examined gender differences in response distortion. A pilot study by Stein and colleagues (2002) measured response distortion among adolescent smokers, and found no significant differences between the genders. However, the sample size was quite small (n = 51) and warrants caution in the interpretation of results. Clearly, there is a need for further research on the extent of response distortion tendencies in girls and boys.

Several study limitations are noteworthy. We focused only on Caucasian boys and girls, so it is still an open question as to how gender may impact the PEI's psychometric properties in different gender/ethnic subgroups. Also, the study was limited to only English-speaking adolescents. Finally, we did not directly address whether gender-specific content may be absent from the PEI. Any test's external validity is compromised to the extent that it is not measuring constructs or characteristics that are relevant to populations for which the test was intended. Thus, the PEI may be limited in its use across genders if certain gender-specific content is not adequately addressed.

REFERENCES

Barkley, R., Fischer, M., Edelbrock, C., & Smallish, L. (1990). The adolescent outcome of hyperactive children diagnosed by research criteria, I: An 8-year prospective follow-up study. *Journal of the American Academy of Child and Adolescent Psychiatry, 29,* 546-557.

Biederman, J., Wilens, T., Mick, B., & Faraone, S. (1997). Is ADHD a risk factor for psychoactive substance use disorders? Findings from a four-year prospective follow-up study. *Journal of the American Academy of Child and Adolescent Psychiatry, 36,* 21-29.

Cady, M., Winters, K.C., Jordan, D., Solberg, K., & Stinchfield, R. (1996). Motivation to change as a prediction of treatment outcome for adolescent substance abusers. *Journal of Child & Adolescent Substance Abuse, 5,* 73-91.

Crowne, D.P. & Marlowe, D. (1960). A new scale of social desirability independent of psychopathology. *Journal of Consulting Psychology, 24,* 349-354.

Dakof, G., Tejeda, M., & Liddle, H. (2000). Predictors of engagement in adolescent drug abuse treatment. *Journal of the American Academy of Child and Adolescent Psychiatry, 40,* 274-281.

Guthmann, D.R. & Brenna, D.C. (1990). The Personal Experience Inventory: An assessment of the instrument's validity among a delinquent population in Washington State. *Journal of Adolescent Chemical Dependency, 1,* 15-24.

Hawkins, J., Catalano, R., & Miller, J. (1992). Risk and protective factors for alcohol and other drug problems in adolescence and early adulthood: Implications for substance abuse prevention. *Psychological Bulletin, 112,* 64-105.

Henly, G.A. & Winters, K.C. (1988). Development of problem severity scales for the assessment of adolescent alcohol and drug abuse. *The International Journal of the Addictions, 23,* 65-85.

Henly, G.A. & Winters, K.C. (1989). Development of psychosocial scales for the assessment of adolescent alcohol and drug abuse. *The International Journal of the Addictions, 24,* 973-1001.

Hsieh, S. & Hollister, C.D. (2004). Examining gender differences in adolescent substance abuse behavior: Comparison and implications for treatment. *Journal of Child & Adolescent Substance Abuse, 13,* 53-70.

Jainchill, N., Yagelka, J., Hawke, J., & De Leon, G. (1999). Adolescent admissions to residential drug treatment: HIV risk behaviors pre- and post-treatment. *Psychology of Addictive Behaviors, 13,* 163-173.

Johnston, L.D., O'Malley, P.M., & Bachman, J.G. (2001). *Monitoring the Future national survey results on drug use, 1975-2000, Vol. 1: Secondary school students* (NIH Publication No. 01-4924). Bethesda, MD: National Institute on Drug Abuse.

Johnston, L.D., O'Malley, P.M., Bachman, J.G., & Schulenberg, J. (2005). *Monitoring the Future national survey results on drug use, 1975-2004, Vol. 1: Secondary school students* (NIH Publication No. 05-5727). Bethesda, MD: National Institute on Drug Abuse.

Kahler, C., Read, J., Wood, M., & Palfai, T. (2003). Social environmental selection as a mediator of gender, ethnic, and personality effects on college student drinking. *Psychology of Addictive Behaviors, 17,* 226-234.

Latimer, W., Winters, K.C., Stinchfield, R., & Traver, R. (2000). Demographic, individual, and interpersonal predictors of adolescent alcohol and marijuana use following treatment. *Psychology of Addictive Behaviors, 14,* 162-173.

Leccese, M. & Waldron, H. (1994). Assessing adolescent substance use: A critique of current measurement instruments. *Journal of Substance Abuse Treatment, 11,* 553-563.

Opland, E., Winters, K.C., & Stinchfield, R. (1995). Examining gender differences in drug-abusing adolescents. *Psychology of Addictive Behaviors, 9,* 167-175.

Rahdert, E. (Ed.) (1991). *The Adolescent Assessment/Referral System Manual.* Rockville, MD: U.S. Department of Health and Human Services, ADAMHA, National Institute on Drug Abuse, DHHS Pub No. (ADM) 91-1735.

Raniseski, J. & Sigelman, C. (1992). Conformity, peer pressure, and adolescent receptivity to treatment for substance abuse: A research note. *Journal of Drug Education, 22,* 185-194.

Stein, L.A., Colby, S.M., O'Leary, T.A., Monti, P.M., Rohsenow, D.J., Spirito, A., Riggs, S. & Barnett, N.P. (2002). Response distortion in adolescents who smoke: A pilot study. *Journal of Drug Education, 32,* 271-286.

Substance Abuse and Mental Health Services Administration. (2005). *Results from the 2004 National Survey on Drug Use and Health: National Findings* (Office of Applied Studies, NDSDUH Series H-28, DHHS Publication No. SMA 05-4062). Rockville, MD.

Weinberg, N.Z., Rahdert, E., Colliver, J.D., & Glantz, M.D. (1998). Adolescent substance abuse: A review of the past 10 years. *Journal of the American Academy of Child and Adolescent Psychiatry, 37,* 252-261.

Winters, K.C. (2003). Screening and assessing youth for drug involvement (pp. 101-124). In J. Allen and M. Colombus (Eds.), *Assessing Alcohol Problems: A Guide for Clinicians and Researchers (2nd edition).* Rockville, MD: National Institute on Alcohol Abuse and Alcoholism.

Winters, K.C. & Henly, G. (1989). *Personal Experience Inventory Test and Manual.* Los Angeles: Western Psychological Services.

Winters, K.C., Latimer, W., Stinchfield, R., & Egan, E. (2005). Measuring adolescent substance abuse and psychosocial factors in four ethnic groups of drug abusing boys. *Experimental and Clinical Psychopharmacology, 12,* 227-236.

Winters, K.C., Latimer, W., Stinchfield, R., & Henly, G. (1999). Examining psychosocial correlates of drug involvement among drug clinic-referred youth. *Journal of Child & Adolescent Substance Abuse, 9,* 1-17.

Winters, K.C., Stinchfield, R., & Henly, G.A. (1993). Further validation of new scales measuring alcohol and other drug abuse. *Journal of Studies on Alcohol, 54,* 534-541.

Winters, K.C., Stinchfield, R., & Henly, G.A. (1996). Convergent and predictive validity of scales measuring adolescent substance abuse. *Journal of Child & Adolescent Substance Abuse, 5,* 37-55.

doi:10.1300/J029v16n01_07

Index

Numbers followed by "f" indicate figures; "t" following a page number indicates tabular material.

Aberdeen Area Adolescent Alcohol and Other Drug Abuse Prevention System (AODAPS), 41-43,42f, 45-46,50

Aberdeen Area Indian Health Services, 41,45
  Division of Field Health, 41

Adolescent(s), SUDs among
  mapping clinical complexities of, typological study of, 5-24. *See also* Substance use disorders (SUDs), adolescents with, mapping clinical complexities of, typological study of
  progress in,1-4
  research related to, 2

Adolescent alcohol use, marijuana use associated with, concordance among objective-, self-, and collateral reports, 53-68
  study of, 55-66,58t-59t,61t
    assessment instruments in, 56-57
    data analysis in, 57
    discussion of, 65-66
    methods in, 55-57
    procedures in, 56
    results of, 57,58t-59t
    subjects in, 55-56
    urinalysis in, 57

Adolescent Diagnostic Interview, 74

Adolescent drug abuse
  measuring of, gender differences in, 91-108. *See also* Personal Experience Inventory (PEI)
  psychosocial factors associated with, measuring of, gender differences in, 91-108. *See also* Personal Experience Inventory (PEI)

Adolescent substance abuse, in Mexico, Puerto Rico, and the U.S., survey formats of, 69-89. *See also* Longitudinal Study of Adolescent Health

Adolescent Substance Abuse Survey, of Rhode Island, 70

Alcohol
  tobacco, and other drug (ATOD) use, 28
  Tobacco, and Other Drug (ATOD) Use by Indiana Children and Adolescents Survey, 70

Alcohol and Other Drug Use Among Students (ESPAD) survey, 71

Alcohol use, among adolescents, marijuana use associated with, concordance among objective-, self-, and collateral reports, 53-68

Alcohol use, among adolescents, marijuana use associated with, concordance among objective-, self-, and collateral reports. *See also* Adolescent alcohol use, marijuana use associated with, concordance among objective-, self-, and collateral reports

American Indian Youth, screening of, for referral to drug abuse prevention and intervention services, 39-52. *See also* Indian Health Service-Personal Experience Screening Questionnaire (IHS-PESQ)

Anderson, T.W., 11

Andrews, V.C., 55

AODAPS. *See* Aberdeen Area Adolescent Alcohol and Other Drug Abuse Prevention System (AODAPS)
Arthur, N., 25

Bachman, J.G., 44
Basic Scales, in PEI, 94-95
Beebe, T.J., 29, 36
Bogenschneider, K., 36
Botzet, A.M., 3,25,91
Brief Symptom Inventory (BSI), 9
Broadening the Base of Treatment for Alcohol Problems, 41
BSI. *See* Brief Symptom Inventory (BSI)
Burleson, J.A., 3,53

Cantwell, D.P., 54,66
CASI. *See Comprehensive Adolescent Severity Inventory (CASI)*
CDC. *See* Centers for Disease Control and Prevention (CDC)
Center for Immigration Studies, 85
Center for Substance Abuse Prevention (CSAP), Western and Central CAPT of, 27,31
Center of Epidemiological Studies Depression Scale (CESD-A), 77
Centers for Disease Control and Prevention (CDC), 78
Centers for the Application of Prevention Technologies (CAPT), Western and Central, of CSAP, 27,31
CESD-A. *See* Center of Epidemiological Studies Depression Scale (CESD-A)
Cigarette use, gender as factor in, 92
Clinical Scales, in PEI, 95
Colon, H.M., 77
Community, described, 26

Community Readiness Model, of Tri-Ethnic Center, 28-29
Community Readiness Survey, of MIPH, 28,30t,31
Comprehensive Adolescent Severity Inventory (CASI), in adolescent substance abuse evaluation, 8-10,19
Cooper, M.C., 11
CSAP. *See* Center for Substance Abuse Prevention (CSAP)
Current Population Survey, 85

Dakof, G., 93
DeWolfe, J., 39
Dillman, 29
DISC–IV. *See* NIMH Diagnostic Interview Schedule for Children–Revised (DISC–IV)
Dishion, T.J., 20
Drug abuse, among adolescents, measuring of, gender differences in, 91-108. *See also* Personal Experience Inventory (PEI)
Drug abuse prevention and intervention services, screening of American Indian Youth for referral to, 39-52. *See also* Indian Health Service-Personal Experience Screening Questionnaire (IHS-PESQ)
Drug Use Among Adolescent Students study, 77-78
design of, 77
participants in, 77
procedure in, 78
survey instrument in, 78
Drug Use Among Adolescent Students survey, 72
Drug Use Frequency (DUF) items, on PEI, 96

Dryfoos, J.G., 26
DUF items. *See* Drug Use Frequency
(DUF) items

Edelbrock, C., 55,66
Edwards, R.W., 35,36
ESPAD survey. *See* Alcohol and Other
Drug Use Among Students
(ESPAD) survey

Fleiss, J.L., 11-12
Floyd, L.J., 69
Frantz, J., 10

Gabrielsen, K.R., 26
Gender
as factor in cigarette use, 92
as factor in measuring adolescent
drug abuse and related
psychosocial factors, 91-108.
See also Personal Experience
Inventory (PEI)
Goodman, 27-28
Graham, D., 39
Grothaus, D., 26

Hagan, T.A., 5,10
Henly, G., 93
Hillery, G.A., 26
Hogan, J.A., 26
Hollister, C.D., 92,105
Hsieh, S., 92,105

IHS-PESQ. *See* Indian Health
Service-Personal Experience
Screening Questionnaire
(IHS-PESQ)

Indian Health Service-Personal
Experience Screening
Questionnaire (IHS-PESQ),
39-52
convergent validity of, 47-48,48t
discussion of, 49-50
factor structure in, 48-49
initial scale development for, 43-45
method of use of, 46, 46t
original psychometrics of, 44-45
procedure for use of, 43-44, 46, 46t
psychosocial risk factors of, 48, 49t
reliability of, 47, 47t
results of use, 46-49, 47t-49t
subjects in, 43,46,46t
Institute of Medicine (IOM), 41
International Longitudinal Survey of
Adolescent Health, 69-89. *See
also* Longitudinal Study of
Adolescent Health
IOM. *See* Institute of Medicine (IOM)

Johnston, L.D., 44,78
Jumper-Thurman, P., 35

Kaminer, Y., 3,53
Kentucky Conference for Prevention
Research, 27

Latimer, W.W., 3,69,93
Leukefeld, C., 27
Liddle, H., 93
Logan, T.K., 27
Longitudinal Study of Adolescent
Health, 69-89
design of, 72
discussion of, 83-86
in Mexico, results of, 79-81,80t
participants in, 72-73,74t
procedure of, 75-76
in Puerto Rico, results of, 81-82,81t

results of, 79-83,80t,81t,83t
substance use frequency in, 75
survey instrument, 73-75
in U.S., results of, 82-83,83t
Luna, N., 26

3-M Parent Collateral Report, 62
9-M Parent Substance Collateral Report,
    60,62
3-M Youth Self-Report, urinalysis and,
    60,61t
Mann-Whitney tests, 32,33
MANOVA, 12
Marijuana use, among adolescents,
        alcohol use associated with,
        concordance among objective-,
        self-, and collateral reports,
        53-68
Marijuana use, among adolescents,
        alcohol use associated with,
        concordance among objective-,
        self-, and collateral reports. *See
        also* Adolescent alcohol use,
        marijuana use associated with,
        concordance among objective-,
        self-, and collateral reports
Marlowe-Crowne Desirability Scale, 95
Marlowe-Crowne Social Desirability
    Scale, 44
Maryland Adolescent Survey, 70
McDermott, P.A., 5,10
McNemar's test, 57
Medina-Mora, M.E., 69,76
Mexico, adolescent substance abuse in,
        survey formats of, 69-89. *See
        also* Longitudinal Study of
        Adolescent Health
Meyers, K., 5,10
Milligan, G.W., 11
Mills, J., 36
Minnesota Adolescent Health Survey, 73

Minnesota Institute of Public Health
    (MIPH), Community Readiness
    Survey of, 25-38. *See also*
    MIPH Community Readiness
    Survey
MIPH. *See also* Minnesota Institute of
    Public Health (MIPH)
MIPH Community Readiness Survey,
    25-38
    analysis in, 32
    discussion in, 34-36
    introduction to, 26-29
    measures in, 29-30,30t
    methods in, 29-32, 30t
    procedure in, 31-32
    rater agreement in, 32-33,33f
    results of, 32-34,33f,34t
    sample in, 29
    scale norms in, 33-34,34t
Monitoring the Future (MTF) survey,
    70,71,78-79,86,92
    data analysis plan in, 79
    design of, 78
    participants in, 78
    procedure of, 79
    survey instrument in, 78-79
Moscoso, M.R., 77
MTF. *See* Monitoring the Future (MTF)

National Institute of Health annual
    survey of drug use, 96
National Survey of Drug Use, 72,76-77
    design of, 76
    participants in, 76
    procedure of, 77
    survey instrument in, 77
NIMH Diagnostic Interview Schedule
    for Children–Revised (DISC–
    IV), 9

Oakes, J.M., 85-86
O'Brien, M.S., 69

O'Donnell, D., 55
Oetting, E.R., 35
Oja, P., 26
O'Malley, P.M., 44
Opland, E., 92

Parent Collateral Report
  urinalyses and, 60,62
  Youth Self-Report and, 62-63
Parent Collateral T-ASI, Youth T-ASI
  Substance subscale and, 63
  urinalyses and, 62
Parent-Youth Alcohol associations, 63
Paronen, O., 26
Parrilla, I.C., 77
Partnership for a Drug Free America
  community survey, 55
PCA. *See* Principal Component Analysis
  (PCA)
PEI. *See* Personal Experience Inventory
  (PEI)
Pentz, 27
Perlman, M.D., 11
Personal Experience Inventory, 73,75
Personal Experience Inventory (PEI),
  44,91-108
  Basic Scales in, 94-95
  Clinical Scales in, 95
  described, 93
  discussion of, 104-106,105t
  DUF items on, 96
  factor analysis in, 103,104t
  internal consistency of, 99,100t
  measures in, 94-95
  method of, 94-98
  participants in, 97-98
  PICS in, 95
  Problem Severity Scales in, 94-95
  procedure for use of, 98
  psychometrics of, 96-97
  Psychosocial Scales in, 95
  reliability of, 99-100,100t
  response distortion in, 103
  results of, 98-104, 99t-102t
  temporal stability of, 99-100
  validity of, 101-103,101t,102t,104t

Personal Experience Screening
  Questionnaire (PESQ), 42-43
  psychometrics of, 43-45
  revision and validation of, for use in
    AODAPS, 45-46
Personal Involvement with Chemicals
  Scale (PICS), in PEI, 95
PESQ. *See* Personal Experience
  Screening Questionnaire
  (PESQ)
Peyrot, M., 27
PICS. *See* Personal Involvement with
  Chemicals Scale (PICS)
Plested, B., 35
PRIDE Drug Survey, 70
Principal Component Analysis (PCA),
  103
Problem Severity Scales, in PEI, 94-95
Psychometrics, of PEI, 96-97
Psychosocial factors, adolescent drug
  abuse–related, measuring of,
  gender differences in, 91-108.
  See also Personal Experience
  Inventory (PEI)
Psychosocial Scales, in PEI, 95
Puerto Rico, adolescent substance abuse
  in, survey formats of, 69-89.
  See also Longitudinal Study of
  Adolescent Health

Q-sort, 31,32

Randall, M., 10
Research, on adolescent substance abuse,
  2
Rhode Island, Adolescent Substance
  Abuse Survey of, 70
Rios-Bedoya, C.F., 69
Robles, R.R., 77

Sechrist, R.A.J., 25
Sharma, A., 25,26
Smith, H.L., 27

Smitham, D.M., 35
St.Cyr, W., 39
Stein, L.A., 106
Stinchfield, R., 91,92,93
Substance abuse, among adolescents. *See*
    Adolescent substance abuse
    progress in, 1-4. *See also*
    Adolescent(s), substance abuse
    among, progress in
Substance use disorders (SUD),
    adolescents with, mapping
    clinical complexities of,
    typological study of, 5-24
CASI in, 8-9
clinical implications of, 19-21
discussion of, 19-22
external criterion variables in, 9
introduction to, 6-8
measures in, 8-9
method in, 8-12
participants in, 8
procedure in, 10-12
profile components in, 9
research implications in, 21
results of, 12-19,13t-18t
typal development in, 10-11
typal discrimination in, 16-19,18t
typal explication in, 12,15-16,15t-17t
typal stability in, 11-12
typal structure in, 12-15,13t,14t
Substance use disorders (SUDs), youth
    with, assessment of, 54,55
SUDs. *See* Substance use disorders
    (SUDs)

Teen Addiction Severity Index, in study
    of concordance among
    objective-, self-, and collateral
    reports of marijuana use
    associated with adolescent
    alcohol use, 56
Tejeda, M., 93
Tri-Ethnic Center, Community
    Readiness Model of, 28-29
T-TASI change from baseline, 63-64
T-tests, 32

United States (U.S.), adolescent
    substance abuse in, survey
    formats of, 69-89. *See also*
    Longitudinal Study of
    Adolescent Health
United Way of America, 27
University of Minnesota, 97
University of Minnesota Institutional
    Review Board, 72
Urinalysis
    9-M Parent Substance Collateral
      Report and, 60,62
    3-M Youth Self-Report and, 60, 61t
    Parent Collateral T-ASI, 62
    in study of concordance among
      objective-, self-, and collateral
      reports of marijuana use
      associated with adolescent
      alcohol use, 57
    Youth T-ASI Substance subscale and,
      60

Vasquez, M.A., 69
Velez, M., 77

Wandersman, 27-28
Ward, J.H., Jr., 10-11
Webb, A., 5, 10
Weissman, M.M., 55,66
Williams, K., 27
Winters, K.C., 4,25,39,55,66,91-93

Youth Risk Behavior Surveillance
    Survey (YRBSS), 70
Youth Self-Report, Parent Collateral
    Report and, 62-63
Youth T-ASI Substance subscale
    Parent Collateral T-ASI and, 63
    urinalysis and, 60
YRBSS. *See* Youth Risk Behavior
    Surveillance Survey (YRBSS)

BOOK ORDER FORM!

Order a copy of this book with this form or online at:
http://www.HaworthPress.com/store/product.asp?sku= 5971

Adolescent Substance Abuse
New Frontiers in Assessment

___ in softbound at $20.00 ISBN-13: 978-0-7890-3506-6 / ISBN-10: 0-7890-3506-5.
___ in hardbound at $40.00 ISBN-13: 978-0-7890-3505-9 / ISBN-10: 0-7890-3505-7.

COST OF BOOKS _____

POSTAGE & HANDLING _____
US: $4.00 for first book & $1.50
for each additional book
Outside US: $5.00 for first book
& $2.00 for each additional book.

SUBTOTAL _____
In Canada: add 7% GST. _____

STATE TAX _____
CA, IL, IN, MN, NJ, NY, OH, PA & SD residents
please add appropriate local sales tax.

FINAL TOTAL _____
If paying in Canadian funds, convert
using the current exchange rate,
UNESCO coupons welcome.

❏ **BILL ME LATER:**
Bill-me option is good on US/Canada/
Mexico orders only; not good to jobbers,
wholesalers, or subscription agencies.

❏ **Signature** _____

❏ **Payment Enclosed: $**_____

❏ **PLEASE CHARGE TO MY CREDIT CARD:**
❏ Visa ❏ MasterCard ❏ AmEx ❏ Discover
❏ Diner's Club ❏ Eurocard ❏ JCB

Account #_____

Exp Date_____

Signature_____
(Prices in US dollars and subject to change without notice.)

PLEASE PRINT ALL INFORMATION OR ATTACH YOUR BUSINESS CARD

Name

Address

City   State/Province   Zip/Postal Code

Country

Tel   Fax

E-Mail

May we use your e-mail address for confirmations and other types of information? ❏Yes ❏No We appreciate receiving
your e-mail address. Haworth would like to e-mail special discount offers to you, as a preferred customer.
We will never share, rent, or exchange your e-mail address. We regard such actions as an invasion of your privacy.

Order from your **local bookstore** or directly from
The Haworth Press, Inc. 10 Alice Street, Binghamton, New York 13904-1580 • USA
Call our toll-free number (1-800-429-6784) / Outside US/Canada: (607) 722-5857
Fax: 1-800-895-0582 / Outside US/Canada: (607) 771-0012
E-mail your order to us: orders@HaworthPress.com

For orders outside US and Canada, you may wish to order through your local
sales representative, distributor, or bookseller.
For information, see http://HaworthPress.com/distributors

(Discounts are available for individual orders in US and Canada only, not booksellers/distributors.)

Please photocopy this form for your personal use.
www.HaworthPress.com

BOF06